Holistic Care of the Older Person

Bláthnaid O'Donoghue

BORU

PRESS

Boru Press Ltd
The Farmyard
Birdhill
Co. Tipperary

www.borupress.ie

ISBN 9781916019935
Design by Sarah McCoy
Print origination by Carole Lynch
Illustrations by Andriy Yankovskyi
Printed by GraphyCems Ltd, Spain

A CIP catalogue record for this book is available from the British Library.

For permission to reproduce photographs and artworks, the author and publisher gratefully acknowledge the following:

123RF 127. Alzheimer's Society of Ireland 97. BAPEN 194, 195, 196, 197. Homecare Medical 137. HSE 18. ILO 7, 9. Institute for Further Studies Stockholm 51. Irish Hospice Foundation 152. iStock 29, 30, 184. Shutterstock 6, 41, 43, 45, 47, 69, 75, 81, 95, 118, 143, 151, 154, 178. World Health Organisation 13.

The author and publisher have made every effort to trace all copyright holders, but if any has been inadvertently overlooked we would be pleased to make the necessary arrangement at the first opportunity.

CONTENTS

SECTION 1

THE AGEING PROCESS

IN THIS SECTION YOU WILL LEARN ABOUT:

+ Factors that influence ageing

+ Global trends in ageing

+ Personal and social attitudes to ageing

+ The role of the healthcare professional in promoting positive awareness of the ageing process

+ Ethnic and cultural influences on the older person

+ Challenges and opportunities for the older person

+ Preparing and planning for retirement

+ The importance of nutrition and hydration for the older person

+ The various body systems affected by the ageing process

+ Holistic care and various models of healthcare

chapter 1

AGEING AND AGEING TRENDS

The ageing process is inevitable. It is a time-related action: as we grow older, we age. Ageing is one of nature's most phenomenal wonders. Intrinsic processes occur that contribute to the unique care needs of older people. However, each person will age differently, influenced by several factors. This has an impact on individual well-being, and this is why individualised care is so important when caring for older people.

Culturally, in Ireland older people are cared for by a family member or relative if this is practicable. Home care allows an older person to remain in their own home for longer and home care support services act as a great support to family carers. Alternatively, older people may reside in a nursing home if they have complex care and social care needs.

The issue of long-term care of a family member can be difficult for all concerned, and it can lead to family division and friction and/or to feelings of resentment in the older person. It is important that healthcare professionals attempt to create a home away from home for the older person residing in a community or residential care setting.

Different cultures have different traditions and customs regarding the care of older people. Sub-Saharan Africa has a population of 46 million people, and this number is set to more than triple to 165 million by 2050. (WHO, 2019.)

Culturally, in sub-Saharan Africa older people are cared for in their own homes by younger generations of their family who often have little support or training. Within this setting, women and girls are often seen as being the primary caregivers and the duty of care mostly falls on the female population. The World Health Organization (WHO) global strategy and action plan on health and ageing identifies that there are challenges faced by countries around the world in responding to the long-term care needs of their ageing populations.

(WHO, 2017.)

> **Reflection**
>
> Reflect on some factors that influence ageing.

Factors That Influence Ageing

There are many factors that affect the ageing process and these differ for each individual. Some older people remain active and physically healthy; they have good mental health and they feel connected to and respected by their community. They could be described as having 'aged well', and they have a strong sense of well-being. Others do not 'age well': they have physical and/or mental health challenges, which contributes to inactivity and reduced participation in the community or other networks.

The factors that influence ageing can be broken down into **external factors** and **internal factors**. We can further categorise these factors into biological, mental, behavioural, nutritional and socio-economic factors.

External factors

Improvements in the last century in the areas of nutrition, hydration, hygiene, sanitation, housing and access to healthcare have had a positive impact on the ageing process. Other factors include where an individual lives, socio-economic status, level of education, occupation, access to health insurance and income.

Other external factors that influence an individual's well-being as they age include level of physical activity, alcohol consumption, smoking status and polypharmacy (the large use of medication without a review of their use).

Internal factors

Internal (or biological) factors such as genetic background, disease, characteristics and inherited traits also affect the ageing process. Body composition, physical disability, auditory or visual impairment, pain and dental health can also impact our ability to age well. Our gender can also influence how we age.

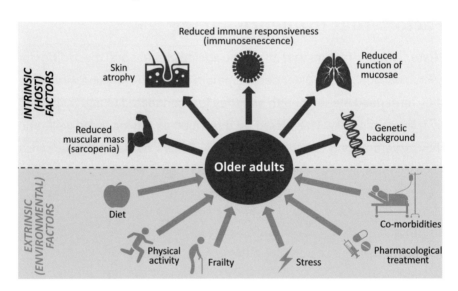

Growth and Ageing

Ageing is a complex process. The majority of countries have accepted the chronological age of 65 years as a definition of 'elderly' or an older person. Interestingly, there is no United Nations (UN) standard numerical age distinction, although they have agreed that 60-plus years is acceptable in relation to the definition of an older person. However, we must remember that age is only a number and that our age does not define who we are, our abilities or our inabilities.

(WHO, 2002.)

There are many scientific hypotheses as to how and why we grow old, including cell damage, which causes our bodies to malfunction. Another theory is that because our DNA is linear, each time one of our cells divides, a piece of the chromosome is lost, and it is the depletion of cells that leads to cellular ageing and disease.

Moreover, as we age, our metabolic rate slows down. This means that the chemical reactions that keep our bodies alive slow down; our cells therefore become less efficient and this affects the functioning of our vital organs. Another change is a reduction in the elasticity of our muscles, joints and ligaments, which can result in a loss of dexterity and agility. It can also lead to stiffness and pain in our joints.

Some elderly people will notice changes to their posture and gait (manner of walking). The skeleton provides support and structure to the body. Joints enable the skeleton to be flexible, facilitating movement. Within a joint, bones do not directly touch each other. They are cushioned by cartilage, synovial membranes and fluid. Depletion of the joints may lead to inflammation, pain, stiffness and bone deformities. The effects range from minor stiffness to severe arthritis.

Muscles keep bones in place, providing stability. Assisted by joints, they play an important role in moving the body. Coordination is directed by the brain but is affected by changes in the muscles and joints. Adaptation in the muscles, joints and bones affects our posture and our strength to walk. Muscle fragility can lead to fatigue, weakness and reduced mobility. This increases the risk of muscle contractures (changes or deformities that can cause stiffness when walking) and pressure sores.

People lose bone density as they age, particularly women after menopause. Bones lose calcium and other minerals. They can become

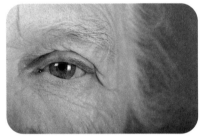

brittle, and the risk of injury increases. Height decreases, mainly because the trunk and spine shorten. Changes occur to our body mass index, which in turn is associated with a loss or 'atrophy' of muscle tissue.

Task Discuss and write down other changes you notice in older age.

Global Ageing Trends

The world's population is ageing. The majority of countries worldwide are experiencing growth in the number and prevalence of older people.

As reported by the WHO and the UN in 2011, 'population ageing is both one of humanity's greatest triumphs and one of its greatest challenges'.

Population ageing is set to become one of the most compelling social revolutions of the twenty-first century, with implications for many sectors within the economy including healthcare, housing, transport and social protection.

(WHO, 2011.)

According to evidence from World Population Prospects in 2019, the number of older people, i.e. those aged 60 years or over, is expected to more than double by 2050 and to more than triple by 2100. This trend will see the population growing from 962 million globally in 2017 to 2.1 billion in 2050 and 3.1 billion in 2100. Without exception, population demographics of those aged 65 years or over are growing faster than all younger demographics.

(Source: https://www.un.org/development/desa/publications/world-population-prospects-the-2017-revision.html)

According to global population estimates by the UN, the number of older people aged 80 or over is projected to more than triple by 2050, from 137 million in 2017 to 425 million in 2050. The proportion and life span of a population are determined by demographic processes to include fertility, mortality and migration.

(UN, 2017.)

Task Can you think of other reasons why people are living for longer?

Task What other changes do you believe can contribute to older people living for longer into the future?

Life expectancy at birth by region, both sexes combined, from 1950 to 2050

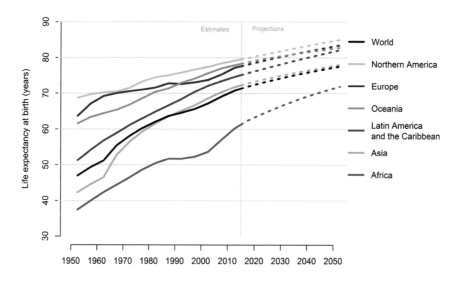

(Data source: United Nations (2017). World Population Prospects: the 2017 Revision.)

According to the WHO, the global population of older people is expected to increase from an estimated 524 million in 2010 to nearly 1.5 billion in 2050.

(WHO, 2011.)

National Ageing Trends

In Ireland, life expectancy tables are produced by the Central Statistics Office (CSO) every five years. The most recent life expectancy table was produced in 2012. In Ireland, the life expectancy for men is 78.4 years and for women is 82.8 years.

(CSO, 2019.)

Task Discuss and write down why you think women have a longer life expectancy than men.

CSO figures released in April 2019 state that the population of the Republic of Ireland reached 4.92 million. A report by the Department of Health on population showed that in 2002, the number of older men was 189,155; in 2021 that figure is set to nearly double. In comparison, in 2002, the number of older women was 246,846; this number is set to increase by 128,989 by the year 2021.

The report highlights that the number of older people living alone will also increase, which is relevant to those providing care to older people. It is predicted that by 2021 there will be 211,000 older people living alone. The north-western counties will have the highest number of older males living alone, while the cities of Dublin, Cork and Limerick will have the highest number of older females living alone.

(Source: www.cso.ie/en/releasesandpublications/er/pme/populationandmigration estimatesapril2019/ Population Ageing in Ireland: Projections 2002–2021, Published: 16 June 2004.)

Task Identify how predicted rates of population ageing in Ireland will impact on the provision of care for older people.

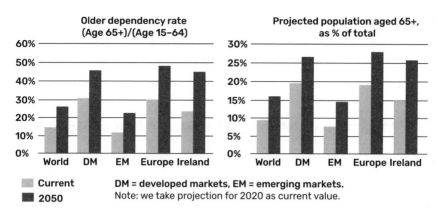

Older dependency rate (Age 65+)/(Age 15–64)

Projected population aged 65+, as % of total

Current
2050

DM = developed markets, EM = emerging markets.
Note: we take projection for 2020 as current value.

(Source: UN Population Division.)

Positive Ageing

The National Positive Ageing Strategy outlines Ireland's vision for ageing and older people. It promotes the view of ageing as a lifelong process, i.e. it is not something that starts on our sixty-fifth birthday; it is shaped by the choices we make from birth. The strategy underlines the importance of older people keeping well and active, and it focuses on opportunities for older people to contribute to society as workers, caregivers and volunteers.

(Department of Health, 2013.)

Life expectancy in Ireland is rising faster than anywhere else in the European Union. In the last census in 2016, this age group (over 65 years) saw the largest increase in population since 2011, rising by 102,174 to 637,567, a rise of 19.1%. The census recorded 456 centenarians, an increase of 17.2% on 2011. Over half a million or 577,171 in this older age group lived in private households, an increase of 19.6%, while those in nursing homes increased by 1,960 to 22,762.

(Source: https://www.cso.ie/en/csolatestnews/pressreleases/2017pressreleases/presss tatementcensus2016resultsprofile3-anageprofileofireland/)

It is predicted that by 2041 that figure will be 1.4 million, representing up to 25 per cent of the total Irish population.

In Ireland people are living into more advanced years. It is estimated that the number of those aged 80 years and over will increase four-fold from 110,000 in 2006 to about 440,000 in 2041.

(Department of Health, 2019.)

Projected population aged 65 years and over, 2016–2051

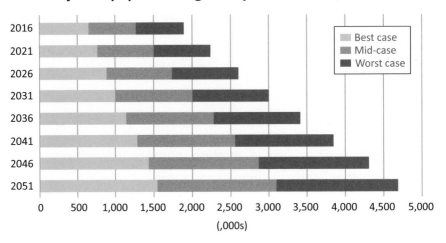

(Source: CSO, Irish Times Graphics, Satuday August 24, 2019.)

Key areas identified in the National Positive Ageing Strategy include:

+ healthy ageing

+ health and personal social services

+ carers

+ employment and retirement

+ education and lifelong learning

+ volunteering

+ cultural and social participation

+ transport

+ financial security

+ housing

+ the built environment

+ safety and security

+ elder abuse.

(Department of Health, 2013.)

Reflection

People are living for longer: how can we use this as an opportunity?

Will older people find new occupations to stay active?

How important is lifelong learning?

How will the needs of older people change?

chapter 2

ATTITUDES TO AGEING, ETHNICITY AND CULTURE

Everyone will have their own personal attitudes to ageing. Some people may have positive attitudes, while others may have negative ones.

> **Reflection**
>
> Reflect on your own attitudes to ageing: are they positive or negative?

Historically, ageing has had negative associations. Older people have been dismissed as being less able than those who are younger. A person's ability to age well can be impacted by personal and social attitudes to ageing. It is very important that healthcare professionals promote positive personal and social attitudes to ageing. In order to do this, we need to be vigilant against ageism and stereotyping.

Negative Attitudes to Ageing

Ageism, stereotyping and discrimination

Ageism can be defined as prejudice or discrimination on the grounds of a person's age. Why does ageism occur? A study carried out by The National Council on Ageing and Older People in 2005 suggests that younger generations allow themselves to see older people differently in order to reduce their own fears and anxieties about ageing. Another theory suggests that it stems from the emphasis placed on youth and physical beauty in western society.

Ageism can have a negative impact on society and on older people. It can make older people feel that they are a burden on society. It can reduce an older person's self-esteem and well-being. It can also be isolating; it can reduce an older person's participation in their local community, and this in turn can negatively impact on services available for older people.

(Department of Health, 2013.)

Stereotyping can also impact the older person's well-being. Stereotyping occurs when fixed beliefs (often negative) are held about a particular group of people. It can lead to the mistaken assumption that all people in that group are the same and that their needs are the same.

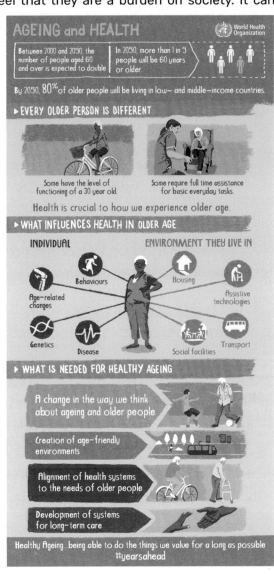

AGEING and HEALTH — World Health Organization

Between 2000 and 2050, the number of people aged 60 and over is expected to double

In 2050, more than 1 in 5 people will be 60 years or older.

By 2050, 80% of older people will be living in low- and middle-income countries.

▶ EVERY OLDER PERSON IS DIFFERENT

Some have the level of functioning of a 30 year old.

Some require full time assistance for basic everyday tasks.

Health is crucial to how we experience older age.

▶ WHAT INFLUENCES HEALTH IN OLDER AGE

INDIVIDUAL
Behaviours
Age-related changes
Genetics
Disease

ENVIRONMENT THEY LIVE IN
Housing
Assistive technologies
Social facilities
Transport

▶ WHAT IS NEEDED FOR HEALTHY AGEING

A change in the way we think about ageing and older people

Creation of age-friendly environments

Alignment of health systems to the needs of older people

Development of systems for long-term care

Healthy Ageing...being able to do the things we value for as long as possible #yearsahead

Task Can you think of any stereotypes that exist about older people?

Stereotypes that exist about older people suggest they are frail, dependent or 'bed blockers'. Stereotyping has decreased in recent times, but many of these attitudes remain.

+ **Age discrimination** occurs when a person is treated differently because of their age. Age discrimination can be direct or indirect.

+ **Direct age discrimination** happens when someone treats you worse than another person in a similar situation because of your age.

   (Source: https://www.equalityhumanrights.com/en/advice-and-guidance/age-discrimination)

+ **Indirect discrimination** can occur when a personal or organisational attitude influences decision-making and the provision of services within a community. An example of an older person being subject to indirect discrimination is if they are not involved in planning their care or reviewing their care plan. This can disempower an older person.

Task Work in pairs and discuss how an organisation might indirectly discriminate against an older person.

Key Points to Remember

+ There is a growing number of people over the age of 65 in Ireland.

+ The ageing process is a natural process.

+ Each person is individual and deserves individualised care.

+ Each person's needs are different and can change on a day-to-day basis.

+ Treating the older person with dignity and respect is key.

+ Ageism and stereotyping can have a negative impact on the older person.

+ It is important that we promote positive attitudes to ageing.

Positive Attitudes to Ageing

Role of the Health Care Assistant (HCA) in promoting positive attitudes to ageing

The WHO defines positive ageing as:

> **The process of developing and maintaining the functional ability that enables well-being in older age.**

Older people require HCAs and other healthcare professionals to adopt a positive attitude to ageing and the ageing process.

Task Working in groups, discuss how you can help to create positive awareness around the ageing process.

Contributions we can all make to promote positive attitudes to ageing

+ Show respect to older people: treat them as you would treat anyone else.

+ Promote choice.

+ Promote inclusion and create awareness of inclusion and the older person.

+ Seek the opinion and contribution of the older person to public policy.

+ Encourage the older person to get involved in their local community. Acknowledge the contribution the person makes.

+ Advocate for the needs of the older person.

+ Do not engage in ageist conversation.

+ Help to de-stigmatise ageing and the ageing process by seeing the positives, not the negatives. For example, challenge beliefs that older people are only sick, frail and that they live in nursing homes.

+ Encourage continued improvements in lifelong learning programmes.

+ Be proud of the job you do when caring for the older person.

+ Speak about and praise the contribution that older people have made to your life.

+ Celebrate your age to help resolve negative beliefs in relation to ageing.

+ Promote Positive Ageing Week and get involved in local initiatives.

+ Promote opportunities linked to ageing such as having more time to explore a new career path, develop new friendships and defy expectations.

Task Investigate Positive Ageing Week and any activities that are run in your area under this initiative.

Note: You're only as old as you feel . . .

In 2016 researchers from The Irish Longitudinal Study on Ageing (TILDA) published a report called 'You're Only as Old as You Feel!' The researchers found that older people with negative attitudes towards ageing had a slower walking speed and worse cognitive abilities two years later, compared to older people with more positive attitudes towards ageing. This was true even after participants' medications, mood, life circumstances and other health changes that had occurred over the same two-year period were accounted for.

This is an important finding about the impact of attitudes to ageing. In conclusion: 'Negative perceptions of ageing may modify the association between frailty and frontal cognitive domains in older adults.'

(Robertson & Kenny, 2016)

Ethnic and Cultural Considerations

We are living in a multicultural world. It is important that health care assistants working in a healthcare system that is diverse and dynamic understand that there are certain ethnic and cultural factors to consider when caring for individuals within various care settings.

Ethnicity

Ethnicity is the act of belonging to a social group that has a common national or cultural tradition. Ethnic groups share history, ancestry, language and geographic origin. Their shared identity exists independently of nationality. For example, communities that identify as being of Irish ethnicity have developed as a result of emigration to countries such as England and the United States.

Inclusion and integration in healthcare

Culture is commonly defined as the bespoke and shared values, beliefs, actions, behaviours and customs of a group of people. Interculturalism is the promotion of understanding and respect between people from different cultural backgrounds. The fundamental principle of interculturalism is the willingness of individuals and organisations to acknowledge and respect cultural diversity.

In order to provide holistic, individualised care to older people, health care assistants must be aware of and support interculturalism. It is vital to remember that each person may hold and follow different aspects of cultural identity including nationality, ethnicity and religious belief, and therefore has a unique set of values and beliefs.

This is important in relation to the provision of personal care and intimate care: we must acknowledge and respect that cultural norms can differ. An understanding of cultural norms and values is particularly important when providing spiritual and end-of-life care.

To learn more about interculturalism in relation to healthcare, consult *Health Services Intercultural Guide,* a document developed and published by the Health Service Executive (HSE) in 2009.

Key Points to Remember

+ Be aware of your own cultural identity.

+ Understand that people of different cultures have different beliefs, ways of communicating, interacting, behaving and responding.

+ Accept and appreciate that cultural and spiritual beliefs impact patients'/residents' health and health-related beliefs, help-seeking behaviours, interactions with healthcare professionals and healthcare practices.

✚ Respond appropriately to patients'/residents' cultural and/or ethnic backgrounds in order to provide them with optimal care in line with best practice guidelines.

Individualised person-centred care is the cornerstone to ensuring the delivery of high-quality healthcare. Everyone deserves to have their cultural and ethnic beliefs upheld and to be treated with dignity and respect in relation to all aspects of their care interventions.

Cultural needs can include:

✚ diet

✚ language: is there a need for an interpreter?

✚ hair care

✚ intimate care

✚ male/female preferences

✚ care interventions, e.g. blood transfusions

✚ religious needs

✚ dress

✚ communication

✚ holistic therapies

✚ alternative medicines.

Task Working in groups, use the *HSE Intercultural Guide* to identify a specific cultural group. Using the guide, investigate how this group's cultural preferences can influence the care you can provide and how it is provided.

Case Study: **Mr H**

Mr H's swallow has been deteriorating, so he takes his tablets with food. The past few mornings, he has been refusing. You are the health care assistant caring for Mr H this morning, and you ask him why he has been refusing his food and his medicines. Mr H informs you that it is Ramadan and he is unable to eat from sunrise to sunset. You inform the other members of the multidisciplinary team that this is the reason why Mr H has been refusing his medicines and his food. It is decided to alter Mr H's mealtimes and medication administration times to ensure that his cultural beliefs are respected while his healthcare needs are met.

It is always useful to take an interest in an older person's beliefs and values. It is good practice to ask an older person about their traditions or customs. Remember: every care intervention should be seen as an opportunity to get to know the person you are caring for and to engage with their social, cultural and psychological needs.

chapter 3

CHALLENGES AND OPPORTUNITIES FOR THE OLDER PERSON

We have learned that there are more people living beyond the age of 65 than ever before. This is a welcome and accepted change in the demographics of Ireland and of countries around the world. Positive attitudes to ageing help older people to feel that they can 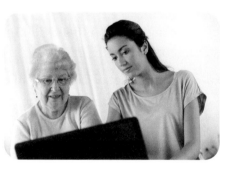 contribute meaningfully to society. However, it is well documented that they can also face many challenges in their everyday lives.

The Positive Ageing Programme was established by the HSE as part of the Healthy Ireland Framework. The aim of the programme is to create a holistic 'whole-of-government' approach to creating positive attitudes towards ageing.

(Source: https://www.hse.ie/eng/about/who/healthwellbeing/our-priority-programmes/positive-ageing)

Challenges Faced by the Older Person

+ Health inequalities: feeling marginalised in society due to healthcare waiting lists and health costs.

✚ Older people have been neglected in clinical trials.

✚ As people age, they become more susceptible to chronic disease.

✚ TILDA data shows that 64.8 per cent of people aged 65 years and over have two or more chronic conditions.*

✚ Transport enables independence, but transport is not always accessible for older people, which, combined with a decrease in mobility, can lead to isolation and social exclusion.

✚ Feeling safe and secure is an important psychological need: reports of older people being targeted by criminality in their own homes can cause anxiety.

✚ Exposure of safeguarding issues and elder abuse can cause anxiety.

✚ Discrimination and ageism can have a negative impact on the dignity and respect of the older person.

✚ Accessible information: having difficulties with accessing information online (e.g. due to lack of computer skills, internet connection, etc.)

✚ Service providers' over-reliance on technology: banking via machine as opposed to meeting a bank clerk; self-service check-outs in shops as opposed to being served by a shop assistant.

✚ Financial worries due to reduced income and pension entitlements.

✚ Changes in social relationships: their children as caregivers; being fearful of retirement due to loss of identity and status within the community.

✚ Death of a spouse or friends, and a decline in their circle of friends.

*(Source: https://tilda.tcd.ie/publications/reports) Irish adults transition to retirement – wellbeing, social participation and health-related behaviours. Findings from The Irish Longitudinal Study on Ageing (TILDA) 2019.)

Research also indicates that there are five key factors that can have an impact on the mental wellbeing of the ageing population:

+ Discrimination
+ Participation in meaningful social and recreational activities
+ Relationships
+ Physical health
+ Poverty

(Mental Health Commission 2019.)

Opportunities for the Older Person

As the population ages, there are opportunities from which older people can benefit. Healthcare professionals have an obligation to examine and support opportunities for older people to live healthy and active lives. The older person's quality of life is key. By engaging with and bringing awareness to the opportunities that are available for the older person we can help to improve a person's self-worth, their personhood and their continued self-development into advancing years.

Task Working in groups, discuss some opportunities that exist for the older person in our society.

Opportunities for the older person include:

+ Engaging in education and lifelong learning can help to reduce the risk of cognitive decline and dementia.
+ Participating in learning can increase knowledge, reduce social isolation and improve a person's quality of life.
+ Engaging in social activities and building positive relationships is beneficial for older people, for example, 'Men's Shed'.

✦ Volunteering can be a positive opportunity for retired people in advancing years.

✦ Generativity (a need to transcend personal interests to provide care and concern for other generations) and having more time to give back to local communities can increase a person's personal satisfaction and contentment with their lives.

✦ Assistive technologies can create opportunities for the older person, i.e. Alexa, the voice-controlled assistant from Amazon.

✦ Developments in technological science can offer opportunities and improvements for Ireland's healthcare provision, e.g. Mario the Robot, a supportive companion for people with dementia.

✦ More time to explore new hobbies and pastimes.

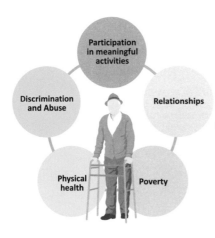

The 5 keys factors that affect the mental health and wellbeing of older people are: discrimination and abuse, participation in meaningful activities, relationships, physical health and poverty.

chapter 4

RETIREMENT

Planning and preparing for retirement can cause mixed emotions for the older person. Our work lives play an important role in keeping both our minds and our bodies active. Often an older person can feel frightened of the prospect of retirement, as they can feel that they are losing a part of their identity, their contribution to society and part of their network of social engagement. These fears can cause anxiety for the older person. The key to overcoming these challenges is to plan and to prepare for retirement.

Preparing and Planning for Retirement

Recent amendments by government to retirement age have extended the age of retirement to 67 years of age. This means that the qualifying age for the state pension will be 67 from 2021 and 68 from 2028. The currently mandatory retirement age is 70 years of age for public sector workers.

The practice of preparing for retirement is important, as people can spend many years of their lives in active retirement. People should start preparing holistically for their retirement in their middle ages. Pre-retirement supports, counselling and education courses are available and can support individuals to plan for their retirement, for example, the voluntary agency Retirement Planning Council of Ireland offer a support network to people preparing for their retirement.

(Source: https://www.citizensinformation.ie/en/employment/retirement/older_people_and_working/retirement_age_in_ireland.html)

The Retirement Planning Council of Ireland is a voluntary agency that was set up in 1974. It has run over 10,730 retirement courses and has helped in excess of 135,500 people to prepare for retirement.

(Source: https://health.gov.ie/wp-content/uploads/2014/03/op_prefs_emp_ret-report.pdf)

Longer Working

As of March 2019, the state pension rate for those aged 66 years and over is €248.30 per week. With an ageing population and with recent changes to the qualifying age for the state pension, many people will want to continue working past the traditional retirement age of 65. The Workplace Relations Commission (WRC) has prepared a code of practice around longer working, setting out best practice for employers on how to engage with employees in the run-up to retirement age.

(Source: https://www.citizensinformation.ie/en/social_welfare/social_welfare_payments/older_and_retired_people/state_pension_contributory.html)

Code of practice on longer working

Some of the measures set out in the WRC's code of practice include:

+ training and education on age diversity and its benefits
+ encouraging the sharing of knowledge between staff
+ highlighting the skill and experience of employees of all ages
+ ensuring that ageism does not exist in policies and procedures
+ developing a culture of appreciating the need for training and development for employees of all ages
+ opening a discussion with an individual about their retirement plans
+ providing supports such as pre-retirement courses or flexible working arrangements

✚ offering counselling and other therapeutic supports to help a person prepare for retirement.

(Source: https://www.mhc.ie/latest/insights/employment-update-guidance-on-working-past-retirement)

If an older person has not prepared or made provision for their retirement they may find it a more difficult transition. This can lead to negative consequences for the older person in relation to their physical, emotional and psychological health.

Healthcare professionals can help older people who are preparing for their retirement by being aware of the various supports that are available and by providing practical information on how to access these supports.

Case Study: Mr Y

Mr Y is 66 years young, and he is hoping to retire in the next few months. He has informed his GP that he is worried about his retirement, and that he feels stressed and is not sleeping. Mr Y has been referred to speak to the practice nurse in the GP's surgery. You are on placement in the GP's surgery: what kind of advice, do you think, will the nurse offer Mr Y?

Task Working in groups, list some common leisure activities chosen by the older person. Then make a second list with some creative recreational ideas that you would recommend to an older person.

chapter 5

NUTRITION AND HYDRATION NEEDS

It is vitally important that the older person's nutritional status is monitored. Nutrition refers to the nutrients that nourish both body and mind, helping to maintain the older person's well-being. Hydration is equally important for the older person; it is important for physical well-being and cognitive health.

A nutritious and well-balanced diet helps to prevent disease, fight infection and promote wound healing. It also supplies us with energy for physical and intellectual activities. When we think of food, we think of it as the fuel that allows us to perform physical and cognitive tasks. As a person ages, this does not change: in fact, there are certain types of nutrients that can help the older person to sustain their cell growth and repair, and to help their immune system to fight infection.

The Food Pyramid

The food pyramid is a universal nutritional template that illustrates the correct portion sizes of foods that we should eat on a daily basis to ensure a balanced diet. It is a universal nutritional template that can help us in relation to monitoring our daily intake of food and fluids.

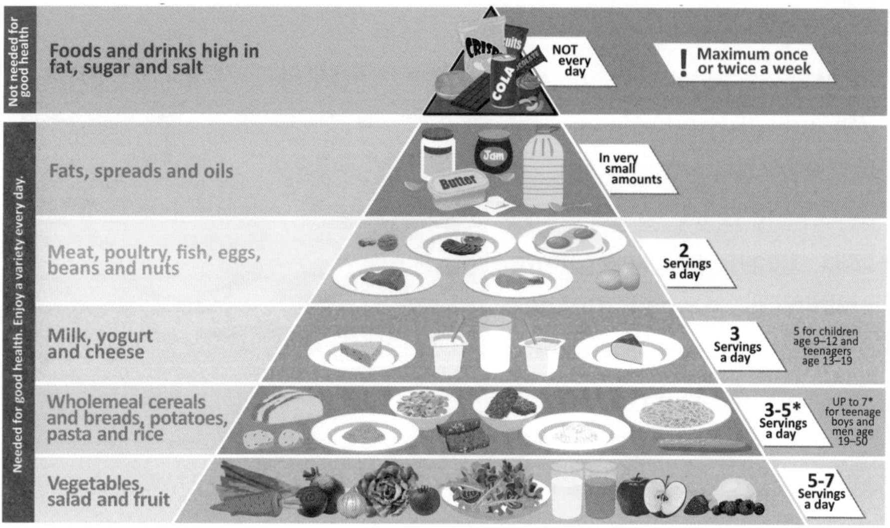
Not needed for good health
Foods and drinks high in fat, sugar and salt
NOT every day
Maximum once or twice a week
Needed for good health. Enjoy a variety every day.
Fats, spreads and oils
In very small amounts
Meat, poultry, fish, eggs, beans and nuts
2 Servings a day
Milk, yogurt and cheese
3 Servings a day
5 for children age 9–12 and teenagers age 13–19
Wholemeal cereals and breads, potatoes, pasta and rice
3-5* Servings a day
UP to 7* for teenage boys and men age 19–50
Vegetables, salad and fruit
5-7 Servings a day

Nutrients

The main nutrients are carbohydrates, proteins, fats, vitamins and minerals. Water is not classified as a nutrient, but it is essential for our survival. Each nutrient has a different function and therefore each one plays an important role in keeping us well into older age.

Carbohydrates

Carbohydrates provide the body with energy. This energy is the fuel that allows our bodies to function and perform our activities of daily living.

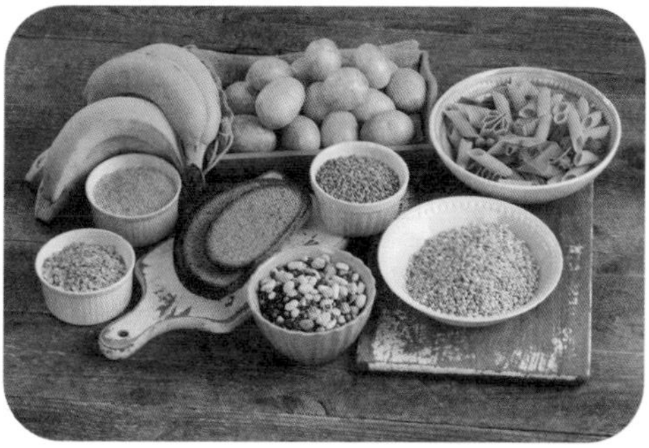

Proteins

Protein is vital for normal cell growth and repair. This is especially important in advancing years: as the body's cells begin to slow down, protein is needed to help maintain normal growth and repair of our cells. Protein forms

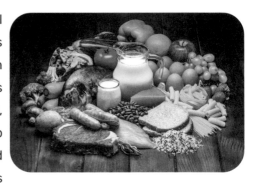

the main part of all cells and tissues, so the body's muscles, organs and immune system are made mostly of proteins.

The older person can become less active with age. This can lead to the circulatory system slowing down, which can compromise skin tissue viability. As a result, they are at risk of developing pressure sores, so protein is a very important nutrient for older people, as it promotes wound healing.

Fats

Fat supplies energy. It also helps to insulate our skin and protects us from heat loss. Too much fat in our diet can lead to health complaints including high blood pressure, high cholesterol, heart disease and obesity. Fat is also important for brain health.

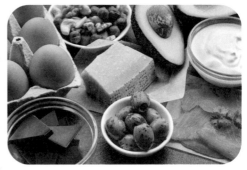

Vitamins and minerals

Vitamins and minerals are vitally important for the body to function properly. For example:

+ **vitamin A** helps to maintain healthy skin, helps vision to adapt to poor lighting and helps to keep our immune system functioning

+ **vitamin D** helps to keep our bones healthy and improves muscle strength

+ **vitamin E** is an antioxidant and is necessary to protect cells from damage

+ **calcium** helps to maintain healthy bones and teeth.

Important Nutrients for the Older Person

Fibre

Eating fibre-rich foods helps to prevent constipation and assists in regular bowel movement. Breakfast can be a good way to get a high-fibre start to the day; for example, add linseed to a wholegrain cereal. Prune juice can also boost fibre intake.

Calcium and vitamin D

Older people need extra calcium and vitamin D to help maintain bone health. Calcium-rich foods include fortified cereals, dark-green leafy vegetables and canned fish with soft bones (like sardines).

Iron and vitamin B12

Iron is responsible for carrying oxygen around the body, while vitamin B12 keeps your brain and nervous system healthy. Many older people do not get enough of these important nutrients in their diet. One of the best sources of iron is red meat, as it is easily absorbed by the body.

Hydration

Water is vital for life, and keeping hydrated is very important for the body to function properly. This is especially important for older people, as dehydration can lead to serious health complications and accounts for a high percentage of all acute hospital admissions.

As we age, our bodies undergo change. The body's metabolic rate slows down, so older people require fewer calories. People over the age of 65 can lose their sense of thirst, and therefore tend not to drink enough. Older people also experience a decrease in appetite: on average, people receive about half their daily water requirement from solid foods including fruit and vegetables, so older people get less fluid from food sources.

Factors that can influence hydration

+ medication

+ exercise

+ behavioural changes

+ emotions

+ environmental changes (if the room temperature is too hot or too cold)

+ weather

+ vomiting

+ diarrhoea.

Dehydration

Dehydration is caused by loss of salts and water in our bodies. It can be caused by severe sweating, extreme heat, excessive urination, vomiting and diarrhoea and certain medications, i.e. diuretic medications. Severe dehydration can be life-threatening to the older person due to the loss of water and salt from the body – there is an imbalance and our vital organs can no longer function properly.

Signs and symptoms of dehydration in the older person

- tiredness
- dizziness
- headaches
- confusion
- change in behavioural/emotional state
- forgetful/disoriented
- lethargic
- low energy levels
- dry mouth
- dry skin
- sunken eyes
- coated and dry tongue
- muscle cramps
- nausea
- rapid breathing
- increased heart rate
- decreased/absent urine output
- poor intake of oral fluids.

Older people will experience the common signs and symptoms of dehydration, including:

| Increased thirst | Fatigue / Lethargy | Dizziness | Headaches | Sticky or dry mouth | Dark or decreased urine output | Loss of skin elasticity | Irritability |

> **Key Point to Remember: Preventing Dehydration**
>
> Prevention is key. Remember: a health care assistant is a constant observer. Even subtle changes to the physical or cognitive health of the person being cared for should be reported in a timely fashion to the nurse/supervisor. Little changes can soon escalate to bigger problems, so be mindful of the signs and symptoms outlined above when attempting to prevent an older person from becoming dehydrated. If left untreated, dehydration can quickly cause severe problems, which can result in death.

Consequences of dehydration for the older person

✚ Change in emotional state: can cause stress and distress

✚ Can be a contributing factor to a person displaying unresponsive behaviour towards you

✚ Confusion

✚ Falls

✚ Urinary tract infections

✚ Delirium or an acute state of confusion due to an infection

✚ Pressure ulcers

✚ Invasive care interventions, e.g. use of artificial hydration, or a urinary catheter to monitor urinary output

✚ Death.

Prevention of dehydration in the older person

To prevent dehydration, it is imperative that the older person is encouraged to drink plenty of fluids during the day. Sometimes it may be necessary to maintain an intake and output chart (see Appendix 1) to monitor daily intake (oral intake of food and fluids, and artificial feeding, e.g. subcutaneously, intravenously or nasogastrically) and output

(output of bodily fluids including urine, faeces, vomit, sputum and wound discharge, if applicable) within a 24-hour period. By ensuring good care in relation to hydration practices, you can help the older person to maintain good health and improve their quality of life. It is also important to educate older people and their caregivers in relation to the importance of staying hydrated.

Constipation

Constipation can be a problem for the older person. Its causes include lack of mobility or a decrease in mobility; a side-effect of medication, particularly for individuals who are taking pain medication (opioids); poor dietary intake; low amounts of fibre in the diet.

The importance of fibre

- Fibre is an indigestible form of carbohydrate.

- Individuals who have low amounts of fibre in their diet can have problems with waste elimination, constipation and haemorrhoids (painful swollen veins in the anus and lower rectum, caused by straining due to constipation).

- Individuals who have diets high in fibre have been shown to be at a decreased risk for obesity, high cholesterol and heart disease.

- Fruits, vegetables, and whole-grain products all contain high amounts of fibre.

Malnutrition

If an older person does not receive the appropriate amount and types of food and fluids, they become malnourished. Malnutrition can be broadly described as a state of insufficient intake of nutrients which can cause weight loss and other adverse effects on the body, the body's functions and clinical well-being.

Nutritional risk screening

In 2009, the Department of Health and the Department of Children and Youth Affairs published guidelines on food and hydration care in hospitals. They recommended that a nutritional risk screening be carried out for every patient within 24 hours of admission to a hospital or residential care setting. The screening is typically carried out by a nurse, however a health care assistant may be asked to record an accurate weight of the person they are caring for.

To help eliminate the risk of malnutrition within clinical care settings, the Health Information Quality Authority (HIQA) outlined the following guidelines in their document 'The National Standards for Safer Better Healthcare':

+ all adult inpatients must be screened for malnutrition, using a validated tool (such as 'MUST')

+ accurate weights must be recorded

+ mealtimes must be protected (no visiting is allowed during specific mealtimes set out as per local policy).

'MUST' (Malnutrition Universal Screening Tool) is a five-step screening tool to identify adults who are malnourished, at risk of malnutrition (undernutrition), or obese. It also includes management guidelines which can be used to develop a care plan. (See Appendix 2.)
(HIQA, 2016a.)

HIQA monitors the nutrition and hydration of patients in Irish hospitals against the 'National Standards for Safer Better Healthcare'.
(HIQA, 2012.)

Assisting an Older Person at Mealtimes

An older person may need assistance at mealtimes due to a decrease in dexterity or cognitive function. Always ensure that you respect the dignity of the older person at mealtimes. You should explain, using a step-by-step approach, that it is a mealtime. Ask the older person if you can assist them, involve them in their care, give them a choice in relation to the menu options, and take your time.

Here are some factors to be aware of:

+ Implement protected mealtimes, as per local policy.

+ Follow therapeutic diets, as per the advice of the multidisciplinary team.

+ Be alert for food allergens, sensitivities and intolerances.

+ Plan mealtimes: do you need any equipment, for example, a clothing protector? If so, always get consent before applying it.

+ Do not rush: allow enough time to support the older person.

+ See mealtimes as an opportunity to engage with the older person and as a social activity.

+ Observe: do you notice any issues with swallow or oral intake, oral hygiene or dental needs?

+ Document dietary and fluid intake.

+ Report any concerns immediately to your supervisor.

Nutrition in Clinical Practice

+ **Presentation:** food, including therapeutic and modified consistency diets, should always be presented in a manner that is attractive and appealing to the older person in terms of texture, flavour and appearance, in order to maintain appetite and nutrition.

+ **Sensory cues:** visual, verbal, sensory and physical cues can all promote independence. Sensory cues, especially those involving smell, can let the person know it is time to eat. This can be particularly useful for those living with dementia.

+ **Social aspect:** mealtimes are 'unhurried social occasions', i.e. an opportunity to communicate, engage and interact with the residents. (Regulatory guidance on food and nutrition requirements for residential services for older people.)

  (HIQA, 2017.)

+ **Food/fluid charts:** older people entering residential care should have their food and fluid needs assessed using a food diary/chart in the first week after admission, and this should be monitored regularly. (See Appendix 1.)

+ **Accurate recording:** remember, food and fluid charts are only as useful as the information documented on them. Exact quantities should be accurately recorded, for example, a spoonful, a forkful or more. The volume of fluids should also be documented in millilitres. Food and fluids refused should be monitored. Records of the food provided for residents are also documented.

+ **Nutritional supplements:** oral nutritional supplements can be used as a treatment for malnutrition in the residential care setting. **NB:** oral supplements must not replace meals.

  (HIQA, 2017.)

Care in Practice

It is useful to remember that an older person being cared for may have a swallowing difficulty. **Dysphagia** is a medical term used to describe a change to or deterioration in a person's ability to swallow food and fluids safely. Always check with the nurse and consult the person's care plan before assisting a person with food or fluid, as some older people may require a modified diet and/or fluids. (See Appendix 3.)

Key Points to Remember

+ Food and fluids should be easy to access for the older person.

+ Adequate amounts of food and fluids should be provided.

+ A nutritional assessment should be performed on admission and regularly thereafter.

+ Be mindful of the amount of assistance a person needs.

+ Assist the person at mealtimes but remember to promote independence.

+ Ensure the type of modification and type of food and fluids provided are appropriate.

+ Record the amount of fluid a person takes in and outputs from their body over a 24-hour period on the Intake/Output chart.

+ Offer drinks using assistive aids if required, for example, a beaker or a straw.

+ Observe for oral health and denture care.

+ Monitor for swallowing difficulties.

+ Report any concerns immediately to a supervisor.

chapter 6

CHANGES TO BODY SYSTEMS IN OLDER AGE

Task Working in groups, write down all the changes you imagine can happen in older age.

As we grow older, we may notice signs of ageing – some more obvious than others. The older person's bodily systems also go through changes as the body ages.

The Musculoskeletal System

The musculoskeletal system provides support and stability for the body and facilitates movement. It consists of the skeleton, muscles, cartilage, tendons, ligaments, joints and other connective tissue that supports and binds tissues and organs together.

Changes to the system as the body ages

+ Muscle mass and strength declines.

+ Muscle atrophy occurs.

+ Walking speed can slow down as a result of all of the above changes.

+ Gait can become unsteady.

+ Coordination and balance can be affected.

+ Loss of height and posture can occur.

+ There is an increased risk of falls and injury as a result of all of the above changes.

The Nervous System

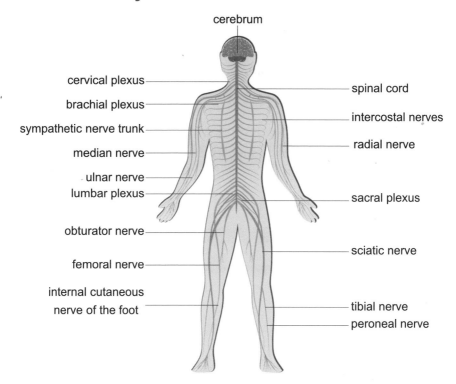

cerebrum

cervical plexus — spinal cord
brachial plexus —
sympathetic nerve trunk — intercostal nerves
median nerve — radial nerve
ulnar nerve —
lumbar plexus — sacral plexus
obturator nerve — sciatic nerve
femoral nerve —
internal cutaneous nerve of the foot — tibial nerve
peroneal nerve

The nervous system consists of a network of nerves and cells that carry messages to and from the brain and spinal cord to various organs in the body. These organs are responsible for controlling the body and for communication among its parts.

Changes to the system as the body ages

+ Short-term memory can decline.

+ Cognitive decline can occur.

+ Bladder control can decline.

+ The ability to learn new things can decline.

+ Reaction time and performance of tasks may become slower, as the brain processes nerve impulses more slowly.

+ There can be a decrease in sensation.

+ Blood flow can decrease.

+ The peripheral nervous system's response to injury is reduced, making older people more vulnerable to injury and disease.

The Circulatory System

The circulatory system is a network consisting of blood, blood vessels and the heart. It supplies tissues in the body with oxygen and other nutrients. It also transports hormones and removes unnecessary waste products.

Changes to the system as the body ages

+ The pumping action of the heart slows down; as a result it becomes less effective.

+ Less blood is pumped to the major organs, causing circulatory problems.

+ The ability to sustain a high level of exercise for a long period of time can decline.

+ The heart's natural pacemaker can lose cells, so the heart can slow down and the individual may develop an abnormal heart rate.

+ The chambers of the heart can fill and empty more slowly, pumping less blood into circulation.

The Digestive System

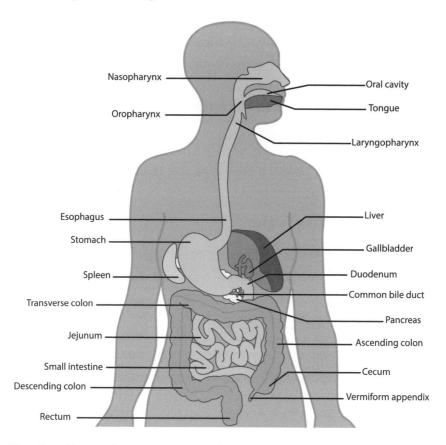

The digestive system breaks down food into smaller components, which can be absorbed and assimilated as nutrients into the body. It includes the gastrointestinal tract, the tongue, salivary glands, pancreas, liver and gallbladder.

Changes to the system as the body ages

+ The stomach cannot contain as much food due to decreased elasticity.

+ The digestion of food becomes less effective and food takes longer to be absorbed.

+ Muscles in the gut and rectum tire, which can cause constipation.

The Male Reproductive System

The male reproductive system consists of sex organs, i.e. penis, scrotum, testes, epididymis, vas deferens, prostate and seminal vesicles. These play a role in the process of human reproduction.

Changes to the system as the body ages

+ Sperm production decreases.

+ Erectile dysfunction can occur.

+ Testicular mass decreases.

+ Testosterone decreases.

+ Prostate gland enlarges, causing slow urination and ejaculation flow.

Female Reproductive System

The female reproductive system is made up of internal and external sex organs, i.e. vagina, cervix, endometrium, ovary, uterus and fallopian tubes. The main function is reproduction.

Changes to the system as the body ages

+ Menopause occurs.

+ Ovaries stop making the hormones oestrogen and progesterone.

+ Ovaries stop releasing eggs.

+ There is an increased risk of bone loss (osteoporosis).

+ There is loss of tone in the pubic muscles, resulting in the vagina, uterus or the bladder falling out of position (prolapsed).

The Respiratory System

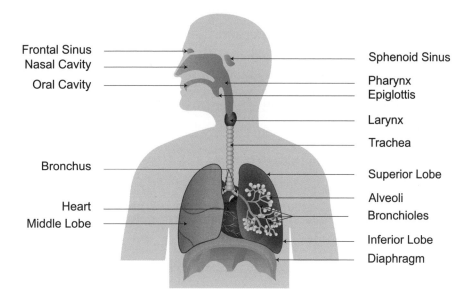

Frontal Sinus
Nasal Cavity
Oral Cavity

Sphenoid Sinus
Pharynx
Epiglottis
Larynx
Trachea

Bronchus

Superior Lobe
Alveoli
Bronchioles

Heart
Middle Lobe

Inferior Lobe
Diaphragm

The respiratory system consists of organs and structures: the airway, the lungs and the muscles of respiration, used for gas exchange. The airway, which includes the nose, mouth, pharynx, larynx, trachea, bronchi and bronchioles, carries air between the lungs and the body's exterior.

Changes to the system as the body ages

+ The respiratory muscles become weak.

+ The lungs lose their elasticity.

+ Less air can be inhaled.

+ Breathlessness can occur.

+ Older people are at higher risk of developing pneumonia (infection of the lungs).

The Integumentary System

This system comprises of the skin and its appendages. These protect the body from damage and water loss.

Changes to the system as the body ages

+ The skin loses its elasticity.

+ The skin becomes thinner and saggier.

+ Wounds become slower to heal.

+ Nails and hair thin.

+ There is a reduction in the amount of natural oil in the skin, resulting in drier skin.

+ There is a decrease in sweat and an increase in intolerance to extremes of heat.

+ There is a decrease in collagen and elastin, which causes the skin to wrinkle.

The Immune System

The immune system is a defence system comprising many biological structures and processes that protect against disease.

Changes to the system as the body ages

+ The ability to protect against infection decreases as immunity decreases.

+ T cells attack disease-causing pathogens: as you age you make fewer T cells, weakening your response to infection.

+ Fewer white blood cells are produced, which limits your ability to fight infection.

The Urinary System

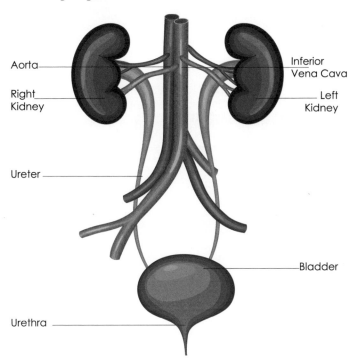

The urinary system consists of the kidneys, ureters, bladder and urethra. Its purpose is to eliminate waste from the body, regulate blood volume and blood pressure, control levels of electrolytes and regulate blood pH.

Changes to the system as the body ages

✚ Arteries bringing blood to the kidneys become narrow; kidney size decreases.

✚ The maximum volume of the bladder decreases.

✚ Muscles in the bladder weaken, which can cause incontinence.

✚ The bladder does not empty fully, leaving some urine behind, which can cause infection.

Other physiological changes to note when caring for the older person

+ There is a loss of pigmentation: hair goes grey.

+ There is a decline in visual acuity: cataracts or glaucoma.

+ Hearing declines.

+ Balance can be negatively affected.

+ Reduced oral cavity size leading to poorly fitting dentures.

+ Gum disease and loss of teeth.

+ Senses can be affected, especially taste and smell.

HOLISTIC CARE AND COMMUNICATION

IN THIS SECTION YOU WILL LEARN ABOUT:

+ The holistic needs of the older person

+ Varying dependency levels and their importance

+ Individual and person-centred care planning

+ Active ageing and strategies to help the older person to age actively

+ Communication skills required to work with the older person

+ The role of the HCA in the practice of holistic care

+ The role of assistive technology to improve the older person's quality of life

chapter 7

HOLISTIC CARE

Determinants of Health

Before we define and examine the importance of holistic care, we should be aware that external factors such as economic, environmental and social inequalities can determine people's risk of becoming ill, their ability to prevent sickness, or their access to effective treatments.

These social health factors have been explored by researchers using several models, but the most widely used is the Dahlgren–Whitehead Rainbow Model. This model maps the relationship between the individual, their environment and health. Individuals are placed at the centre and surrounding them are the different layers of influences on health such as the social and economic environment, the physical environment and the person's individual characteristics and behaviours. The individual comes with a set of fixed genes, however, the influences on health that surround the individual are not fixed and can be modified. The first layer of influences relates to personal behaviour and ways of living that can promote or damage health, such as choosing to smoke or not, eating habits, alcohol use, etc. Individuals are also affected by friendship patterns and the norms of their community.

The next layer is social and community networks, which provide mutual support for members of the community in certain conditions, but they can also provide no support and as such have a negative effect on the individual.

The third layer includes structural factors such as housing, working conditions, access to services and provision of essential facilities, and education.

It is important to be aware of these determinants before you attend to the holistic needs of the older person.

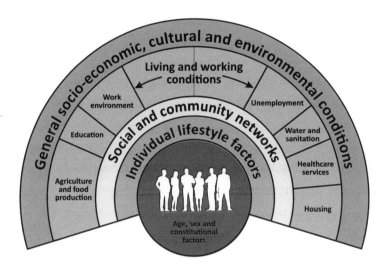

(Source: Dahlgren G, Whitehead M. (1991). Policies and Strategies to Promote Social Equity in Health. Stockholm, Sweden: Institute for Futures Studies.)

Holistic Care

Holistic care incorporates care of the whole person. Holistic care of the older person involves taking care of their physical, emotional, social, psychological and spiritual needs. For example, when you are providing care to the older person, you may help them with their personal care needs, such as a shower or a bed bath. In doing so, you are providing physical care to meet a physical need. However, it is important to remember that every care interaction is an opportunity to meet that individual's holistic needs. For example, you may ask them how they are feeling today; you may offer a compliment to meet their emotional needs; you may chat to the person about the local news or what social events are happening in the area at this time. In such ways you will help to meet their social needs.

The Bio-Psychosocial Model

The bio-psychosocial model is a model of healthcare that incorporates the link between the body, the mind and socio-environmental factors. This approach strives to adopt the benefits of providing holistic and person-centred care.

Healthcare professionals must remember that individuals being cared for have individual needs. One care plan is not suitable for all service users. As you enter work experience, you will learn that each person you care for will have their own uniqueness, their own individual needs and their own set of dynamic circumstances: this is what makes us intriguing as human beings. This approach is set out in line with national best practice and regulatory standards set by HIQA (see Chapter 19).

The bio-psychosocial model of health

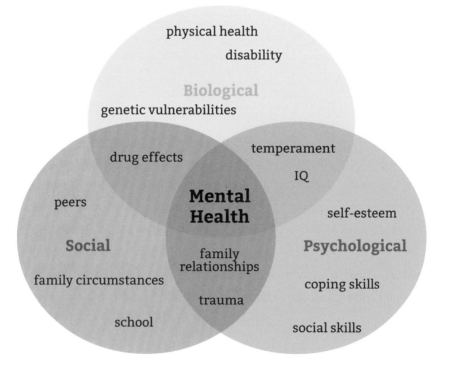

When using the bio-psychosocial model when providing care, it is useful to be aware of the importance of person-centred care also: person-centred care ensures that the person you are caring for is the epicentre of all care interventions performed. The older person should feel in control of their care, and they must be involved in the decision-making process surrounding their care.

Key Points to Remember

+ Confidentiality: the person in receipt of care has the right to have all aspects of their care treated as private and confidential information. All persons (patients/residents/clients/service users) are entitled to the basic right to have confidential information concerning them and their care restricted to those who have a need or a right to know this information.

+ What you hear and what you see within any healthcare setting stays within the parameters of the healthcare environment.

+ Confidentiality preserves dignity and privacy, ensures physical and emotional safety, prevents exploitation and increases client–carer rapport.

+ When writing assignments, always remember to protect the privacy of your client and their care setting. **Tip:** it can also be useful to tell your teacher/corrector that you will use a fictitious name to protect the identity of the person you are caring for.

The 12 activities of daily living

Activities of daily living (ADL) are everyday tasks that a person will perform to thrive. They can also be used as a measurement of a person's functional ability. There are 12 activities of daily living.

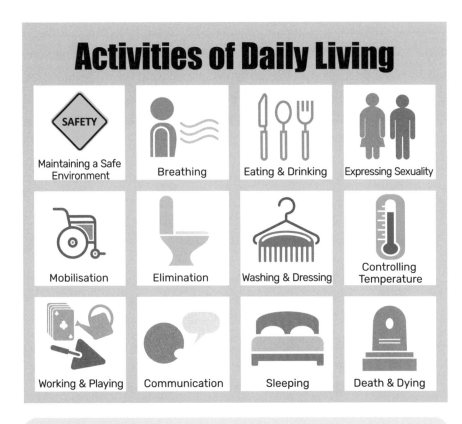

Activities of Daily Living

- Maintaining a Safe Environment
- Breathing
- Eating & Drinking
- Expressing Sexuality
- Mobilisation
- Elimination
- Washing & Dressing
- Controlling Temperature
- Working & Playing
- Communication
- Sleeping
- Death & Dying

Case Study: Mr X

(Using the Bio-pyschosocial model of care)

Mr X has recently been admitted to his local nursing home. He appears to be transitioning well into his new environment. Mr X had a fall at home, and he suffered a broken hip and a broken wrist. Mr X now requires assistance with his activities of daily living including: washing and dressing, elimination, mobilising and maintaining a safe environment. Mr X is an independent man and staff are aware of the importance of promoting his independence. Mr X loves to communicate and interact with staff and residents. He enjoys taking part in the activities within the nursing home and he especially enjoys receiving visits from his family and friends.

Task You are the health care assistant supporting Mr X with his activities of daily living this morning.

✚ How can you assist him with his activities of daily living whilst promoting his independence?

✚ How can you promote Mr X's dignity and respect when providing care?

Case Study: Background Information from Mr X's Care Plan

Biological

Mr X has been living independently at home for the last five years. Mr X has had no recent health complaints. Mr X had suffered from low blood pressure and he had reported feeling dizzy at times. Mr X suffered a collapse at home and, on investigation in the hospital, low blood pressure was found to be reason for his fall, which caused him to sustain his injuries.

Social

Mr X is a very sociable and outgoing gentleman. He is very involved in his local community and loves to attend sporting activities. He is especially interested in GAA: he played for his local club for over twenty years, and he enjoys attending club and county football and hurling games. He also volunteers with his local Tidy Towns committee. He is a member of the local choir and of his local Men's Sheds association.

Mr X has a good family network: his wife passed away almost five years ago, but he receives regular visits from his children (he has two sons and one daughter). His three grandchildren love to visit also. Mr X had previously visited the nursing home to perform with the choir and he knows some of the nursing home residents. He likes to attend the day room so that he can engage with his peers.

Psychological

Mr X reports that he has coping skills, as he had to learn these skills when his wife passed away. He is aware that he is receiving convalescent care within the nursing home and has accepted that currently he would be unable to manage independently at home.

Mr X has been educated on the importance of adhering to the exercise plan that has been planned specifically for him by the physiotherapist. Mr X is keen to work on this exercise plan to help to improve his recovery and his mobility. Mr X also likes to use his iPad to look up information online in relation to his injury to help improve his recovery. All the staff within the nursing home are aware of the importance of setting realistic goals for Mr X's recovery in order to help improve his self-esteem. Mr X's care plan is reviewed regularly by staff.

Task Working in groups, highlight the biological, social and psychological aspects of care that are factors in providing person-centred and holistic care for Mr X.

chapter 8

HOLISTIC NEEDS OF THE OLDER PERSON

As we learned in Chapter 7, holistic care incorporates care of the whole person. The holistic needs of the older person do not necessarily differ from the needs of any other age profile in our society: we all have needs. They include:

+ physical needs
+ emotional needs
+ social needs
+ psychological needs

+ financial needs
+ recreational needs
+ intellectual needs
+ spiritual needs.

Maslow's Hierarchy of Needs is a useful tool that we can use to identify the unique needs of each person.

Maslow's Hierarchy of Needs

Maslow's Hierarchy of Needs is a motivational theory used in psychology, depicted as hierarchical levels within a pyramid. The foundation of the theory is that the lower needs in the pyramid must be met before we can satisfy needs higher up in the hierarchy.

The bottom of the pyramid identifies our most basic needs, for example, food and water. The top of the pyramid identifies more complex self-actualisation needs, for example, the need for a person to achieve their full potential. Once we meet our basic needs on the bottom level of the pyramid, we are inspired and motivated to reach the next level of the pyramid.

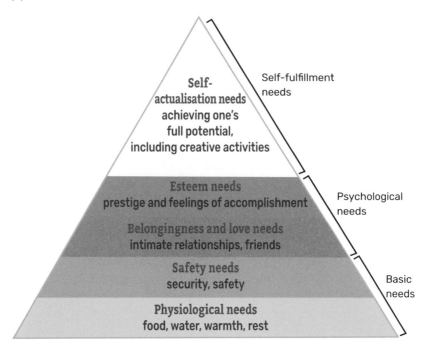

Physiological Needs

This is the lowest level on the pyramid, including our most basic needs for survival. These needs must be met before we can move further up the pyramid. This applies to everyone, regardless of age. Food, drink, shelter, warmth, sleep and response and treatment of illness and injury are fundamental to survival. When providing care to the older person, physical needs are needs that caregivers focus on. This is important, as these needs are the building blocks for meeting needs on all the other levels. However, remember that time spent meeting physical needs also provides an opportunity to assess and meet needs from other levels, for example, esteem needs.

> **Reflection**
>
> Remember to view every interaction or care intervention as an opportunity to engage with and provide intellectual stimulation to the older person. For example, when assisting an older person with washing and dressing, always protect their dignity and respect their safety needs. To meet the person's esteem needs, ask them what they would like to wear and compliment their appearance.

Safety Needs

Once physical needs have been met, an individual moves further up the pyramid, which identifies safety and security needs. The elderly, particularly those who may be vulnerable due to physical, cognitive or intellectual impairment, need and deserve to feel secure and safe. Safeguarding the older person is paramount to protect them from abuse or neglect within their own home or any care environment.

All adults should be given the opportunity to engage in positive risk-taking within their own environment, so it is essential that staff do not engage in over-use of restrictions and restrictive practices.

Care providers have a big role to play in creating a safe and secure environment for the older person. Assessing risk is important, but in doing so it is important to remember that the older person is an adult, so they should be treated as an adult, regardless of individual circumstance or cognitive decline. Sensitivity is needed when considering risk in relation to a person's safety needs, for example, when identifying and discussing concerns around driving, management of a person's own medication, cooking or living independently. When a care intervention is taken to safeguard the older person, they may react to the loss of their independence. It is useful to include the person in their care plan so that they feel in control and safe in their environment.

Social Needs

The ability to connect and engage socially is of vital importance for everyone, not least for the ageing population. The ability to form and maintain relationships is just as important in older age as it is in the developmental stages. Friends and social relationships are needed from the cradle to the grave. The ability to form and preserve trusting relationships is crucial to prevent the older person from becoming isolated in society.

The need to engage intergenerationally is also very important: the older person can provide learning and wisdom to younger generations, whereas younger generations can also provide learning and improve the quality of life of the older person. Similarly, intimacy and social interactions are important in older age, so the older person should be given the opportunity and privacy to express these needs. Having frequent visits from family, friends, caregivers and peers can help to meet the older person's social and recreational needs.

Self-Esteem Needs

The older person has the right to feel recognised and appreciated for their ideas, abilities and continued contribution to society. As a person ages, they can lose their sense of self-worth due to illness, disability or deterioration in cognitive ability. The loss of self-worth can be devastating to the older person's well-being and their quality of life. Healthcare professionals have the opportunity to add to the lives of those they are caring for by incorporating all aspects of a person's holistic care needs to help increase an individual's self-esteem needs; for example, getting to know a person's history, their values and their beliefs can help to encourage the person to feel recognised and appreciated. Showing a genuine interest in a person's life story and their pastimes can improve their esteem needs.

Examples of ways to boost an older person's self-esteem needs include helping them to write a diary, construct a family album or record stories and events from their life. Activities like this can help an older person to reflect on their achievements and their abilities, which in turn can increase their self-esteem and give them a sense of purpose.

Other considerations to remember when helping to meet a person's self-esteem needs include: providing dignified and respectful care; recognising achievements and promoting independence; and recognising and appreciating their reputation, their status within society and their individual prestige.

Self-Actualisation Needs

The highest level of Maslow's Hierarchy of Needs is the need for self-actualisation. Self-actualisation occurs when a person realises their own individual potential and continues to seek further personal growth. The need of self-actualisation helps the individual to realise that their life's journey is just as important as their destination. As the older person has a wealth of life experience and maturity, they should be encouraged to reach self-actualisation. Healthcare professionals can help an older person to achieve this need by recognising that they have a continued desire to fulfil their dreams and ambitions: a person's aspirations do not become stagnant just because they are ageing. Engaging in lifelong learning and education, volunteering, joining new organisations and taking on new hobbies can help an older person to continue to reach their personal goals.

Key Points to Remember

+ Each older person is of worth and value.

+ Each older person possesses a broad range of abilities and needs.

+ Each older person has unique physical, psychological, social and spiritual needs.

+ The older person and his/her family/representative are the unit of care. It is important for the older adult's family or their named representative to be involved in the individual's care plan and they must be informed regularly of the needs and the plan of care for the older person, as well as any changes to their condition.

+ The older person and their family have the right to make informed decisions about all aspects of their care.

(Source: Nursing and Midwifery Board of Ireland [NMBI], 2015.)

chapter 9

DEPENDENCY LEVELS

Each older person you will care for will have different needs and different levels of need. This means that some older people will require assistance with all their activities of daily living, whereas others will require less assistance or limited supervision. This is described as their dependency level. It is useful to remember the 12 Activities of Daily Living so that we can reflect on the needs of the older person in relation to their individual everyday tasks.

Task Can you list the 12 Activities of Daily Living?

The Barthel Scale

An assessment tool called the Barthel Scale (Mahoney & Barthel, 1965) is used to measure performance in relation to a person's ability to self-perform their activities of daily living and can therefore be used to determine an older person's level of dependency. The scale (see Appendix 4) uses ten variables describing a person's activities of daily living and their mobility. These variables are scored: a high score is associated with a high level of independence and therefore a greater likelihood of the person being able to live and care for themselves; a lower score identifies a person as being less independent, so that person will usually require a higher level of care. The amount of time and physical assistance (number of care staff) required to care for a person can be identified using this tool.

The tool looks at these ten variables:

+ presence or absence of faecal incontinence

+ presence or absence of urinary incontinence

+ help needed with grooming

+ help needed with toilet use

+ help needed with feeding

+ help needed with transfers (e.g. from chair to bed)

+ help needed with walking

+ help needed with dressing

+ help needed with climbing stairs

+ help needed with bathing.

When this assessment tool is used to identify an individual's dependency level, we can classify those we care for into three categories: high dependency, medium dependency and low dependency.

High dependency	Based on the individual profile of the older person, he or she will require the assistance of at least two people for all their activities of daily living
Medium dependency	Based on the individual profile of the older person, he or she will require the assistance of at least one to two people for all their activities of daily living
Low dependency	Based on the individual profile of the older person, he or she will require the assistance/supervision of at least one person for all their activities of daily living.

Person-Centred Care

Person-centred care is a necessity to provide effective, efficient, high-quality healthcare to the older person. In the working world, it will be rare that you will ever meet two people with the exact same background, set of circumstances or care needs: this is why the provision of person-centred care is crucial. Person-centred care places the individual and their needs at the centre of the care you provide. It means adapting your skillset to provide high-quality holistic healthcare to meet the unique and individual needs of each older person. It is vital that the older person is included in any decision-making in relation to their care and in the implementation of the care that is provided.

The care plan

An individual's care needs and how to fulfil those care needs will be documented in an individual care plan. Quite simply, a care plan can be defined as a written document that tells a healthcare professional how to provide holistic care for an individual based on the individual's needs and preferences. It is good practice to seek information about a person's care plan and their needs before you provide any care intervention.

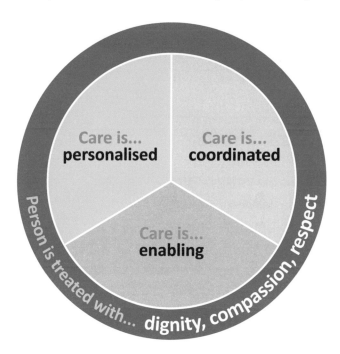

HIQA outlines that person-centred care is one theme that must be met to be in line with their national standards, 'A Guide to the National Standards for Safer Better Healthcare'. Theme 1, 'Person-Centred Care', outlines that healthcare professionals should respect the values and dignity of each person for whom they provide care. In a person-centred care service, healthcare professionals actively listen to all service users and support them to be involved in their own care and to have a voice in relation to how the healthcare service is run.

(HIQA, 2012.)

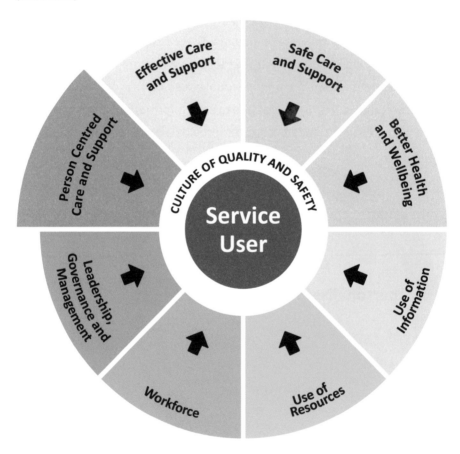

Maintaining Low Dependency Levels with Active Ageing

A report by TILDA found that:

✚ More than half (53 per cent) of older people in Ireland volunteered at some time within a one-year period, 17 per cent doing so at least once per week.

✚ Retired older people who frequently volunteer have been found to have a better quality of life and fewer depressive signs and symptoms.

✚ Sixty per cent of the older population take part in active and social leisure activities at least once per week.

(Ward, 2019.)

Active ageing is associated closely with social participation. As highlighted in the National Positive Ageing Strategy, a crucial feature of successful ageing is that we consider the contribution of older people beyond their contribution to their family: older people are important participants in improving local communities and contributing actively to community-based organisations and clubs.

(Department of Health, 2013.)

Many adults volunteer their time and experience to organisations that operate within the community to the benefit of society. Moreover, volunteers also benefit personally in a number of ways, including improved physical, psychological and social well-being. Many older people also participate in a wide range of other recreational activities, including attending educational and lifelong learning classes, participating in sports, fitness and exercise and socialising in pubs and restaurants.

Families can benefit from having grandparents care for their children when needed, but how does caring for a grandchild affect the grandparents' quality of life? According to a recent TILDA study, research indicates that quality of life is higher for those who cared regularly for their grandchildren among those aged 65 to 74 years and those aged 75 years and over, compared to those who have grandchildren but do not care for them on a regular basis.

Older people also contribute substantially to the well-being of younger generations, both their children and grandchildren. Older people can also provide financial transfers to their children and grandchildren: the rising cost of childcare in Ireland can preclude parents from returning to work, so grandparents who provide childcare can enable many parents who have pre-school-aged children to remain in the labour market.

(Department of Health, 2013.)

chapter 10

COMMUNICATING WITH THE OLDER PERSON

Good communication is an important part of the healing process. It is necessary to have effective communication skills to care for the older person, as it is crucial that they understand your verbal and non-verbal communication, and equally that you understand and respond appropriately to theirs. Remember: communication is much more than the words we speak.

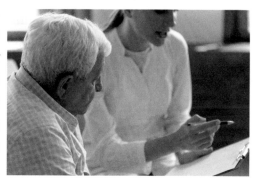

Task Working in groups, discuss the importance of communication when caring for the older person. List communication challenges that you may encournter when providing care for the older person.

Communication is important to everyone: it is essential to have our needs met, for example. It can also be the basis of forming therapeutic relationships. It is useful to remember that we communicate with our whole body: verbally and non-verbally. Our non-verbal cues include body language, facial expression and tone of voice. The skills needed to provide meaningful and therapeutic communication to the older person are the same skills needed to communicate with any other person.

However, as we age, so does our body and our sensory perceptions, including hearing, sight and touch. It is important to keep this in mind when communicating with the older person.

Health care assistants have a knowledge and an understanding of the ageing process, and often have past experience of caring for older people. This knowledge and experience can influence thoughts and feelings about the older person being cared for. When communicating with an older person, it is important to be mindful of the individual's unique communication needs, for example, does the person have dementia? Does the person require a hearing aid, glasses or any other assistive aid to improve the person's ability to communicate with you?

When you introduce yourself to an older person, it is important that you ask them what they would like to be called, or what name they are known by. Not only are you showing respect to the older person, you are also laying the foundations for forming a trusting and therapeutic relationship with them. Once you get to know the individual needs of the older person, you can determine their communication needs and endeavour to deliver sensitive and compassionate care to them.

Active listening is an important process in relation to communication. 'Listening' requires the healthcare professional to use their senses to get the total message. The healthcare professional will listen with their ears to the words spoken and acknowledge the tone of voice; with their mind to help create an understanding of message; and with their eyes to the language of the body. The healthcare professional must also listen to themselves, i.e. they must note their reaction to the message they have received and the way in which they are coping with it.

Practical Tips for Communicating with the Older Person

+ Introduce yourself.

+ Ask the person how he/she would like to be referred to.

+ Approach from the front.

+ Speak on the side of the 'good' ear if a person has a hearing impairment.

+ Encourage the use of hearing aids or glasses if necessary.

+ Communicate at face level.

+ Do not cover your lips.

+ Reduce or eliminate background noise.

+ Relax.

+ Speak in a low tone: don't shout.

+ Allow time to respond.

+ Speak slowly.

+ Use simple words and short sentences.

+ Avoid using medical jargon.

+ Combine verbal communication with non-verbal and other means of communication.

+ Write things down if necessary.

+ Pay attention to the said and the unsaid.

+ Stop talking and listen.

+ Communicate respect and understanding.

+ Try reminiscence and validation.

+ Use assistive aids to communicate with the older person if they are available, e.g. picture boards, Braille and apps on phones or iPads that have been designed to improve communication with the older person.

YES						NO
Nurse	Doctor	Carer	Walking Frame	Wheelchair		
Medicine	Pills	Bathroom	Bed	Toilet	Bath	Shower
Bedroom	Hot drink	Cold drink	Food	Help	I don't understand	Slippers
Light	Sit up/down	TV	Telephone	Newspaper	Walk	Teeth
Glasses	Clothes	Bag	Walking Stick	Shopping	Cold	Hot
Alone	Husband/Wife	Family	Garden	Noise	Hearing Aid	Watch
Hairdresser	Priest/Vicar	Worried	Pain	Bored	Tired	Angry

Safe Advice

S is for **simplify**. Instead of using medical jargon, use simple expressions that older people are likely to be familiar with and understand.

A is for **assure**. Don't assume all older people have a communication deficit, for example, a hearing or visual impairment. Assure them they matter by communicating with kindness and involving them in the conversation.

F is for **feedback and information**. Help older people to make informed decisions by sharing information in the way they prefer. Writing or demonstrating something can be helpful. The use of whiteboards and picture boards can be useful if a person has a hearing impairment.

E is for **ease** into it. Avoid sharing too much, too quickly. Unfamiliar situations can be overwhelming, so slow down and allow people time to process information. This is important when caring for a person with dementia or any other cognitive impairment.

A is for **acknowledge**. Don't overlook older people: recognise, engage and listen to them.

D is for **discovery**. Just because someone nods their head does not mean they understand you. Ask older people questions to see if they truly comprehend and to show that you are interested in their intellectual needs.

V is for **value**. Avoid using overly friendly terms. Do not speak to the older person as if they were a child, for example, using expressions such as 'good boy' or 'good girl'. This can be seen as abuse. It is crucial that you communicate with the older person as an adult. Respect older people by using their proper name, for example, Mr Smith.

I is for **individualise**. Acknowledge and respect language barriers and be sensitive to one's personhood, their inherent values and cultural beliefs. If required, use the services of an interpreter.

C is for **communicate** (safe communication). Avoid telling people what to do. Instead, ensure you are promoting an older person's independence by asking the person to do what they can for themselves. If a person needs assistance, ensure that you explain, using a step-by-step approach, how you will perform the care intervention.

E is for **empathise**. Try to understand a situation from the older person's perspective. Attempt to put yourself in the person's shoes. Be aware that an older person can feel very vulnerable when they require assistance with their personal or intimate care. Ensure that you communicate with the person during these times, offering support and reassurance. Only expose areas of skin that need to be exposed for care for the shortest period of time. Explain to the older person that you will use a privacy blanket, that the door is closed or locked and that the curtains or blinds are closed. Be sensitive to the situation, potential challenges and needs.

(Source: https://nursing.uc.edu/content/dam/nursing/docs/CFAWD/ LookCloserSeeMe/Module%204_GDST_Reference%20Guide.pdf)

Key Points to Remember

+ Older people deserve and are entitled to be informed and to partake in the decision-making process regarding their care.

+ The older person has a right to be involved in the planning and the delivery of their care and to be informed if there is any change to the delivery of their care.

+ Even if a person has dementia or memory loss, direct your comments and attention to him or her.

+ Be mindful that at the end of life, it is possible that a person can hear what you are saying, even if they appear unresponsive or if their eyes are closed.

+ At all times, it is important that you provide sensitive, compassionate and therapeutic communication to the older person.

chapter 11

THE ROLE OF THE HCA IN THE PRACTICE OF HOLISTIC CARE

In essence, the role of the health care assistant (HCA) in providing holistic care to the older person is to champion their well-being. It is the responsibility of the HCA to ensure that the physical, emotional, social and spiritual needs of the older person are being met. Moreover, the only way those needs can be determined is by getting to know the older person: their needs, their likes, their dislikes, their background, their hobbies, their interests and their personhood. We are all so different, and it is for this reason that individual and person-centred holistic care is provided.

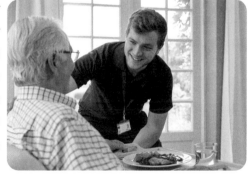

Furthermore, when providing holistic care, it can be useful for the HCA to reflect upon Maslow's Hierarchy of Needs. The pyramid provides us with an overview of the most basic needs to the more complex needs that we have as individuals. When providing care to the older person it is useful to see every interaction as an opportunity for holistic care, i.e. you provide not only physical care, but also emotional, social and spiritual care.

Assessment

You will have to perform a skills demonstration as part of your assessment for this module. Your skills demonstration will be worth 60 per cent of your total mark.

For each type of need below, can you list examples of any other physical, emotional, social, financial, spiritual, religious or safety needs a person in your care may have? Write them in the spaces provided.

Type of need	Examples	Your examples
Physical care needs	+ Assisting a person with a shower, bath or bed bath + Assisting a person with their personal care needs, for example, personal grooming + Assisting a person to the bathroom + Assisting a person with dressing + Assisting a person at mealtimes	
Emotional care needs	+ Asking the person which they would prefer: a shower, bath or bed bath + Asking a person if they have a preference regarding a male or a female staff member assisting them + Involving a person in choosing their clothing by asking them what they would like to wear	

Type of need	Examples	Your examples
Emotional care needs *contd.*	+ Giving a person choice at mealtimes, outlining what is available on the menu and asking what they would like to eat + Complimenting a person's appearance, for example, their hair style or clothing. This can boost a person's self-esteem and promote dignity and respect for the older person, which, in turn, can contribute to a positive emotional or psychological state.	
Social care needs	+ There are opportunities to embrace a person's social care needs while carrying out their physical care needs, for example, asking a person would they like to listen to the radio or to music, or would they like to have the television on in the background. + This is an opportunity for the HCA to interact with and chat to the older person to get to know how they are feeling, if they had any visitors, whether they saw family and friends recently. The HCA could also discuss what's on the news locally, nationally or internationally, for example, was there any local activity on over the past few days in the older person's local environment?	

Type of need	Examples	Your examples
Spiritual care needs	✦ The HCA may need to spend time with an older person to determine their beliefs and help to ensure that their spiritual or religious care needs are being met.	
	✦ Very often in a healthcare setting a priest will visit, and the older person will be given the opportunity to attend Mass, prayers or to speak to the attending priest. The older person may like to be made aware of Mass times, prayer times and any other special events that will be occurring within the setting.	
	✦ The older person may also make the HCA aware of their religious or spiritual beliefs and wishes in the event of something sudden happening, for example, they may like spiritual music playing in the background.	
	✦ Does the older person have a special spiritual connection with music, nature, poetry, writing, or anything else that may help them to feel more relaxed? It is important that the HCA asks these questions as they get to know the older person to ensure that their spiritual needs are being met.	

Key Terms in the Care of Older People

+ **Empowerment:** encourage and promote the older person's ability to perform everyday tasks for themselves.

+ **Advocacy:** speak on behalf of the older person and speak up for their wishes and needs if they are unable to do so for themselves. You are their voice and you promote their interests.

+ **Independence:** engage with the older person when providing care and ensure that they are promoted to do what they can for themselves, for example, ask the older person if they have any limitations and what you can do to support them. It is important to reflect upon their Barthal score, as this assessment helps to determine how much support the older person needs and how much assistance they require with their activities of daily living. **NB:** regardless of the dependency levels of the person you are providing care for, you should always endeavour to promote each individual's independence.

+ **Individualised care:** this means that you are aware that each person has unique needs, that the care you provide is not a one-size-fits-all package, and that you must tailor the care you provide to meet the diverse needs of each person. Good communication skills are needed here so that you can meet the expectations of each person you care for. Getting to know individual needs takes time, and a detailed care plan helps to clarify the individual needs of each person.

+ **Holistic care:** this means caring for the mind, body and soul. Holistic care identifies that an older person's needs go beyond physical care needs; they include emotional, social, spiritual and financial needs too.

+ **Dignity and respect:** dignity and respect are basic human rights. It is vital that each person you care for is treated with dignity and respect. (Dignity is derived from the Latin word *dignitas* meaning 'merit' or *dignus* meaning 'worthy'.)

(Stratton, 2017.)

- Dignity includes not only respecting the person you are caring for, but also respecting that person's right to make their own decisions and choices about matters that affect their life. It is a state, quality or manner worthy of esteem or respect, and (by extension) self-respect.

- **Dignified care:** providing dignified care in any care setting means the care supports and promotes the person's autonomy and self-respect and does not undermine a person's self-respect regardless of any difference. Or, as one person receiving care put it more briefly, 'Being treated like I was somebody'.

  (Help the Aged, 2001.)

- **Choice:** promoting and offering choice to the older person is a very important aspect of providing high-quality care; it provides evidence that you are including the person in the delivery of the care you are providing to them. It also shows that you are treating the person with dignity and respect. HCAs should offer choice to the person in every task that is performed with them, for example, asking a person what they would like to wear when assisting them in getting dressed, or asking them what they would like to eat when assisting them at mealtimes.

- **Self-esteem:** a positive self-image can contribute to a person's self-esteem. If you look good, you feel good. Part of the HCA's role is to provide personal grooming and dressing, so it is important to acknowledge that pride in appearance does not fade with age; people still like to look and feel their best. It is important to ask the older person about their beauty and grooming routine to ensure the person feels good about themselves. It is also important to inspect clothing and footwear to make sure that they are in a good state of repair: if clothing and footwear is becoming worn you should inform your line manager and involve the family also, so that clothing is kept of a high quality.

+ Some other tips to maintain or improve a person's self-esteem are as follows:

  1 Ask the older person for their opinion on their care. Instead of making decisions for them, ask them about the type of assistance they need.

  2 Give the older person tasks to complete. These tasks can be simple tasks such as folding laundry to more complex tasks such as looking after the healthcare setting pet.

  3 Find out what hobbies the person enjoys and set up activities around these hobbies. These hobbies can also improve cognition, intellect and memory, which can help a person to feel better about themselves.

  4 Ask them about their past. Look through photographs with them as they talk about their history. Reminiscence is a very important part of therapy for an older person, especially for those who have dementia. Promoting a person to remember their achievements and life experiences can also improve a person's self-esteem.

+ **Compassion:** compassion can be described as showing genuine concern for the sufferings or misfortunes of others. A healthcare professional's ability to show compassion is a very important interpersonal skill. It is important to attempt to put yourself in the shoes of the individual who may have received bad news or whose health may be deteriorating.

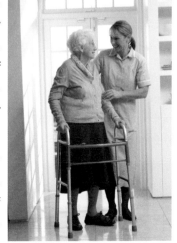

+ **Empathy:** being able to show empathy is not a skill that is learnt, rather it is a component of providing care, where a healthcare professional has the ability to understand and share the feelings of another. This can be difficult, and even though it cannot be learnt, the more exposure a healthcare professional has to difficult situations, the better they might provide compassionate and empathetic care in an honest and sincere way. Empathy is a skill that most healthcare professionals provide without even knowing that they are providing it: it's the listening ear, the gentle touch, the shoulder to lean on. Ultimately, it's the appropriate display of compassion, emotion and interest in the care that you will provide as a healthcare professional.

chapter 12

ASSISTIVE TECHNOLOGY

Assistive technology describes practical aids that are used to improve the quality of life and support the independence of older people and of people living with disabilities. It is:

> **any item, piece of equipment or product system whether acquired commercially, modified or customised that is used to increase, maintain or improve functional capabilities of individuals with disabilities.**
>
> (World Health Organization & World Bank 2011, p.101 World Report on Disability. Geneva, CH; WHO.)

Assistive technology facilitates older people to live in their homes for longer and complete activities of daily living independently. There have been significant developments and innovation in technological science, which offer opportunities and solutions to the health service, its providers and its users. It is important to harness these innovations and optimise their benefits to facilitate healthy ageing.

The "expansion" of Assistive Technology

1980	1990	2000	2010	2020
Medical	Physical Access	Access Software (Some Environments)	Personal (mobile) Devices (all Environments)	Integrated Differentiation

The Benefits of Assistive Technology

✚ Can help people to access their human rights (United Nations Convention on the Rights of Persons with Disabilities 2017)

✚ Provides increased choice, safety, independence and sense of control for the user, which can lead to an improved quality of life

✚ Can reduce burden placed on carers

✚ Can offer improved support for people with long-term health conditions

✚ Offers value for money in terms of user satisfaction and improved quality of life

✚ Can have cost benefits for the health service; for example, Mario the Robot was introduced in care settings in the West of Ireland to help people living with dementia and to help prevent isolation and loneliness.

✚ Facilitates people to get and retain employment

✚ Supports people to remain in their own homes

✚ Supports people to complete their education and/or become digitally literate.

(Enable Ireland & the Disability Federation of Ireland, 2016.)

Mario the Robot

Mario is a robot who talks to the older person, shares the latest news, plays videos and music and reminds the person about everyday tasks. Even though researchers acknowledge that this robot does not replace human contact, they note that it offers support to the older person in an economical way.

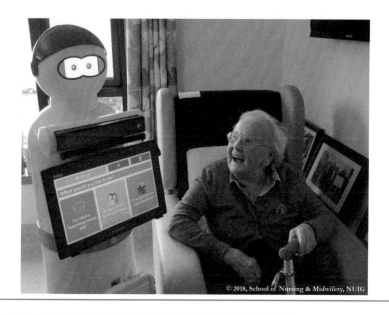

© 2018, School of Nursing & Midwifery, NUIG

Task

+ Investigate the use of assistive technology in the care setting you are working in.

+ Investigate, using online resources, other examples of assistive technology for the older person that may improve their ability to function more independently.

Examples of assistive technologies

✛ Screen-reading software that supports people with vision impairments, as well as those with literacy challenges

✛ Interactive whiteboards

✛ Digitally enhanced audiobooks

✛ Voice-output communication solutions for those who have difficulty with verbal communication

✛ Remote-controlled equipment such as doors, windows and lights, which enable older people to live independently in their own home

✛ Smartphone apps, tablets and iPad devices, which can support the older person to live independently and enhance their quality of life

✛ Wearable technology, which can provide alerts and information. For example, an alert could remind someone to take medication or to leave home at a particular time to catch a bus.

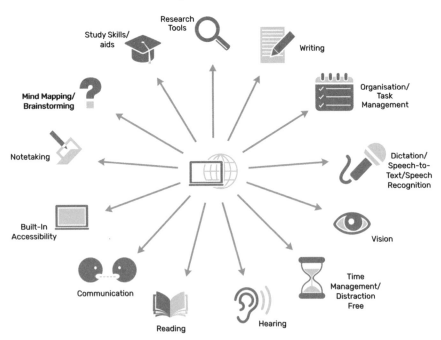

With continued investment in and engagement with assistive technologies by the State, healthcare professionals can support those for whom they care to live independently for longer.

Task Working in groups, discuss and review any other examples of assistive technology you have seen in practice.

Adaptive Technology

Adaptive technology involves any object or system that is specifically adapted for the purpose of increasing or maintaining the capabilities of people with disabilities or frailties, such as limitations to vision, hearing and mobility. It refers to special versions of already existing technologies or tools. Adaptive technologies can help the older person to live more independently in their own environment.

Examples of adaptive technologies

+ Grab bars on bathroom walls for the shower/bath/toilet
+ A raised toilet seat with armrests
+ Non-slip mat for the bath/shower
+ Walk-in showers
+ Stair lifts
+ Walking aids such as walking stick, tripod, walking frame and rollator
+ Reaching/grab aids
+ Hoist-standing/full hoist (note that Patient Manual Handling training is required to use a hoist)

(Source: https://elderlyfallprevention.com/assistive-devices/)

CARING FOR THE OLDER PERSON WITH SPECIFIC NEEDS

IN THIS SECTION YOU WILL LEARN ABOUT:

+ Cognitive and sensory issues that can impact the older person's quality of life

+ Dementia and dementia care

+ Parkinson's disease and holistic care for a person with Parkinson's disease

+ Stroke, stroke rehabilitation and cardiovascular disease

+ Mental illness, including depression and anxiety

+ The impact these conditions can have on the older person, their family members and the multidisciplinary team

+ Applying learning to assessment techniques, using case studies on dementia, Parkinson's disease and stroke

+ Providing holistic care from the perspectives of a Director of Care, a Staff Nurse and a Senior Health Care Assistant through a question-and-answer session

chapter 13

COGNITIVE AND SENSORY ISSUES

In 1946 the WHO defined health as:

> **a state of complete physical, mental and social well-being and not merely the absence of disease or infirmity.**

This definition encompasses the importance of holistic care and can help us to relate to its importance.

(Source: https://www.who.int/about/who-we-are/constitution)

Healthcare professionals in Ireland and all over the world are becoming more aware of specific cognitive and sensory issues in relation to the holistic care of the older person. Cognitive issues generally affect the older person because cognition (our ability to process and understand information) is impacted by a decline in brain health and normal brain function, which is an effect of conditions such as dementia.

It is important to understand the following key terms before learning about some of the individual diseases that can influence the active ageing of the older person.

Key terms

Cognition is the action or process of learning knowledge and understanding through thought, experience and the senses.

Sensory impairment is the impairment of one of the senses (sight, hearing, smell, taste, touch and spatial awareness).

Quality of life refers to the level of well-being of the individual and their degree of satisfaction in relation to a number of human needs.

Chronic diseases are conditions that last one year or more and which require ongoing medical intervention and limit a person's normal activities of daily living.

Chronic Conditions

There are several chronic conditions that can impact the health and well-being and the quality of life of the older person.

Task

+ Working in groups, list five chronic conditions that can affect the health and well-being of the older person.

+ Once you have listed the five chronic conditions, choose one and discuss how this condition can impact the quality of life of the older person.

Chronic conditions that can affect the older person

+ Alzheimer's disease
+ arthritis
+ cancer
+ cardiovascular disease
+ cataracts

+ dementia
+ depression
+ diabetes
+ enlarged prostate
+ glaucoma

- heart attacks
- heart disease
- kidney disease
- lung disease
- macular degeneration
- osteoporosis
- Parkinson's disease
- stroke
- vascular dementia.

When a person is diagnosed with a chronic condition it can have a devastating impact on the individual, their family and their wider circle of friends. An individual can often feel fearful: fearful of the condition and fearful that it will impact their independence and quality of life. It is important that healthcare professionals caring for a person with a chronic condition offer the person continued support, a listening ear and a helping hand. It is particularly important to listen actively to any fears or anxieties the person may have in relation to their care plan.

Reflection

Healthcare professionals will often act as advocates for the individuals they are caring for. Older people can be particularly vulnerable even though they are living well with cognitive decline or a sensory impairment. Verbal and non-verbal dialogue and communication can be helpful to influence and empower the older person living with a chronic condition.

chapter 14

DEMENTIA

Dementia is a term that describes a range of conditions that can cause damage to the brain. This damage affects memory, thinking, language and the individual's ability to perform everyday tasks. Dementia is a chronic progressive problem of cognition, which is failure of the brain's functions.

(The Alzheimer Association of Ireland, 2019).

Dementia can cause a decline in the individual's level of function in memory and cognition and/or a decline in one or more other intellectual functions such as abstract thinking, language or constructional ability (for example, aphasia, apraxia or agnosia). Dementia can also influence a change in personality, e.g. agitation, mood disorder, walking with purpose or exit-seeking behaviour, and depression.

Key terms

Dementia is an umbrella term that describes a number of different diseases, all of which can impact normal brain function and cause cognitive decline.

+ **Aphasia** is an impairment of language, affecting the production or comprehension of speech and the ability to read or write. (National Aphasia Association, 2019)

+ **Apraxia** is a motor speech disorder. The messages from the brain to the mouth are disrupted, and the person cannot move his or her lips or tongue to the right place to say sounds correctly.

- **Agnosia** is the inability to process sensory information; for example, there is a loss of ability to recognise objects, persons, sounds, shapes and smells.

  (Source: https://www.alz.org/alzheimers-dementia/what-is-dementia)

- **Walking with purpose and exit-seeking behaviour** are typical behaviours for many people with dementia, where they seek to find a familiar location, often their own home, the town in which they grew up, an old workplace or a location that holds a strong memory for them. Facilitating a person with the space and freedom to walk with purpose may help that person to maintain their previous enjoyment of walking and exploring. It may allow them to avoid people they don't particularly like, increasing the person's autonomy and sense of control. Afterwards, the individual may have an improved understanding of where they are and their orientation may be improved.

The Dementia Tree

The visual of the trees on the next page gives an understanding of the term: the branches might represent a different type of dementia, such as Alzheimer's disease, vascular dementia, Lewy body dementia and frontotemporal dementia, while the leaves represent brain cells. As the stages of dementia move from early stage to middle stage to later stage, more leaves fall from the tree, representing a progressive decline in the individual's number of brain cells, which will contribute to their cognition, their ability to comprehend everyday tasks and to perform their activities of daily living independently.

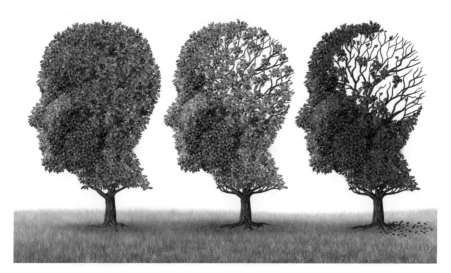

Parts of the brain and their functions

✚ **The parietal lobe:** sensory function, sequence of actions and locating objects

✚ **The frontal lobe:** intelligence, logic, language and personality

✚ **The occipital lobe:** processing information about colour, shape and movement received from the eyes

✚ **The temporal lobe:** memory, attention and verbal language

✚ **The cerebellum:** physical movement and coordination.

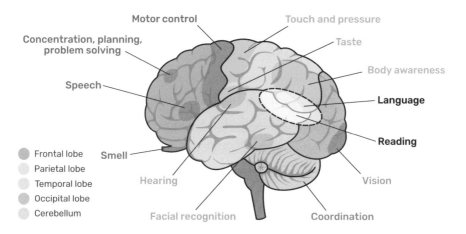

Key Points to Remember

+ Dementia is not one specific disease. It is an umbrella term that describes a wide range of conditions associated with a decline in memory.

+ Dementia is age-related. Its incidence and prevalence increase significantly with advancing years.

+ At the age of 65 years, 5 per cent of people are likely to have dementia.

+ For a person in their nineties, the risk of developing dementia is fifty times greater than that of someone in their 60s.
  (Source: http://dementia.ie/information/what-is-dementia)

+ Dementia (from the Latin *de* meaning 'without' and *mens* meaning 'mind') is a serious loss of global cognitive ability in a previously unimpaired person, beyond what might be expected from normal ageing.
  (Source: https://srcarecenter.com/entity/dementia)

+ Latest figures indicate that eleven people are diagnosed with dementia in Ireland every day.
  (Source: Facts and Figures on https://alzheimer.ie/creating-change/awareness-raising/dementia-in-the-media)

Dementia Statistics

There are currently 55,000 people living with dementia in Ireland. The increase in the number of people living with dementia in the coming years will be significant and could be as high as 132,000 people by 2041, almost three times the estimated number of 47,000 people living with dementia in 2011. (These estimates are based on Census data and population forecasts prepared by the Central Statistics Office.)

Worldwide, the number of people with dementia is currently estimated to be 44 million and is expected to reach approximately 76 million by 2030. (Pierce *et al.*, 2014.)

55,000 PEOPLE ARE CURRENTLY LIVING WITH DEMENTIA IN IRELAND

34,650 WOMEN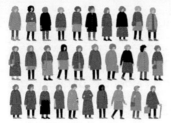

19,800 MEN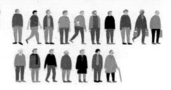

(Source: Dr Suzanne Cahill and Prof Eamon O'Shea, Prevalence and Projections of Dementia in Ireland 2011–2016)

THE AGEING POPULATION IN IRELAND

The population in Ireland aged 65 years and over is projected to increase very significantly from its 2011 level of 532,000 to about 850,000 by 2026.

The very old population (i.e. those aged 80 years of age and over) is set to rise even more dramatically, increasing from 128,000 in 2011 to an estimated 470,000 people in 2046.

(Central Statistics Office, 2013.)

Dementia in numbers

Age Groups	2011	2016	2021	2026	2031	2041
30–59	2,803	2,967	2,982	2,930	2,869	2,686
60–64	1,193	1,303	1,449	1,592	1,696	2,024
65–69	2,734	3,334	3,649	4,069	4,488	5,304
70–74	4,542	5,575	6,868	7,576	8,495	10,141
75–79	7,378	8,328	10,432	12,992	14,467	18,178
80–84	10,924	12,504	14,543	18,632	23,568	30,301
85+	18,319	22,392	27,581	34,131	44,464	71,946
Total	47,893	56,403	67,504	81,922	100,047	140,580

Task   Working in groups, list some of the signs and symptoms associated with dementia.

Signs and Symptoms of Dementia

A person living with dementia may:

+ have difficulty processing information

+ have difficulty finding the right words

+ struggle to remember names, for example, of family or loved ones

+ struggle to recognise people, places and objects

+ struggle to follow direction (verbal instruction/written instruction/prompts/signs)

+ have visual difficulties, for example, judging distances (this can lead to poor mobility, an increased risk of falling, an inability to risk-assess their environment and to maintain a safe environment)

+ experience gradual loss of speech

+ have difficulty eating and sometimes swallowing

+ experience incontinence

+ display exit-seeking behaviour (they appear restless, unable to relax or sit for any period)

+ lose the ability to learn new things

+ forget the immediate past (what happened today or yesterday)

+ perform time- and space-travel, for example, reliving old memories

+ reflect on old memories (positive or negative)

+ lose the ability to follow visual cues (signage/colour schemes)

- ✚ seek out the familiar (life-story books/pictures available to the service user)

- ✚ get stuck on an old, emotional memory track (this can be frightening; it may not always be a positive memory)

- ✚ say whatever they are thinking/lose their inhibitions

- ✚ swear easily.

It is important to note that dementia affects people in different ways. This is representative of the type of dementia and the location of the brain lobe in which brain cell death (neuron-degeneration) has occurred.

Poor or decreased judgment

Frequent memory loss that affects daily activities

Problems with abstract thinking

Problems with language, e.g forgetting simple words

Loss of initiative

Misplacing things or putting them in inappropriate places

Difficulty performing familiar tasks

Changes in personality

Disorientation with time and place

Changes in mood or behaviour

Living Well with Dementia

Life changes when someone develops dementia, but it doesn't end. By understanding dementia, we can help people with dementia to live well. Although there is no cure for dementia, effective help is available and includes:

+ medication and other treatments

+ a range of community supports

+ practical adjustments and adaptations to the person's life and home.

People can live well with dementia through active support from family, friends and the wider community.

(Source: https://www.understandtogether.ie/)

Good dementia care involves using information to develop person-centred care, which is designed to ensure that services are tailored to each individual's circumstances.

> **Residential care staff can determine how best to serve each resident by knowing as much as possible about each resident's life story, preferences and abilities.**
>
> (HIQA, 2016b.)

Concepts of care

Healthcare professionals who provide holistic and person-centred care for the older person living well with dementia should also be aware of the following concepts of care as outlined by HIQA:

+ The provision of person-centred care, including the progression of the disease, memory loss and behavioural/psychological signs and symptoms

+ Strategies for communication to address sensory/cognitive impairment and language barriers

+ A variety of techniques for understanding and approaching the service user who is living with dementia (Guidance on Dementia Care for Designated Centres for Older People, 01 July 2016)

+ An assessment and regular review of the service user's strengths and abilities

+ Division of a person-centred care plan outlining strategies for addressing physical and emotional needs whilst responding effectively to behavioural and psychological signs and symptoms of dementia.

Reflection

A person living well with dementia has an inherent dignity, value and personhood which remains with them throughout the whole course of the disease and should always be respected.

It is important that staff caring for people with dementia see the person, not the condition, that the service user is listened to and that their perspectives and choices are honoured.

Person-centred care for a person living well with dementia

Person-centred care is not just about giving people what they want or providing information, it is about reflecting on people's desires, values, beliefs, family situations, social circumstances and lifestyles, seeing the person as an individual, seeing the world from their eyes and working together to develop appropriate solutions to care needs.

The 'Umbrella Term' of Dementia

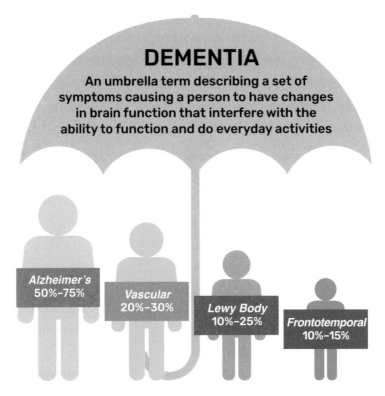

DEMENTIA

An umbrella term describing a set of symptoms causing a person to have changes in brain function that interfere with the ability to function and do everyday activities

Alzheimer's 50%–75%

Vascular 20%–30%

Lewy Body 10%–25%

Frontotemporal 10%–15%

Alzheimer's disease

When a person's brain is affected by Alzheimer's disease, new brain cells stop forming. Furthermore, a process called neuron-degeneration occurs, which means that neurons in the affected person's brain start to change: the neurons' structure and function alter and may even die. The result of this is a shrinking of the brain, called atrophy.

The hippocampus is the centre of learning and memory in the brain. The brain cells in this region are often the first to be damaged. This is why memory loss is often one of the earliest symptoms of Alzheimer's.

Vascular dementia

The second leading cause of dementia is vascular dementia. It accounts for 20 per cent of all cases of dementia. Blood vessels are a fundamental structure for normal brain functioning: they deliver food and oxygen to the brain. Brain function can be damaged if the blood supply to a person's brain is interrupted; this can cause weakening of the blood vessels and can be a contributing factor to a person acquiring vascular dementia.

Neurons stop functioning or die in the part of the brain that was damaged. The resulting symptoms depend on the part of the brain where the stroke happened. Vascular dementia is often the result of multiple strokes that have happened over time.

Lewy body disease

A man named Frederic Lewy examined the neurons of deceased people's brains and found deposits of matter inside the neurons; he later ascertained that these were protein deposits. The protein deposits bind together to form plaques and tangles inside neurons, causing neuron loss and dopamine loss in many brain regions. That is why we can notice symptoms like Parkinson's disease in people affected by Lewy body disease.

Signs and symptoms of Lewy body disease include an altered cognitive decline, which is usually the first symptom to manifest, combined with three additional defining features:

+ pronounced 'fluctuations' in alertness and attention, pronounced drowsiness, lethargy and disorganised speech

+ recurrent visual hallucinations

+ Parkinson's-like symptoms, for example, muscle rigidity and the loss of spontaneous movement.

Frontotemporal dementia

Frontotemporal dementia, which may also be referred to as Pick's disease, is a rare type of dementia. It is believed to be the fourth most common type of dementia. During the early stages, a person's memory may be fine, but their personality, behaviour and language skills can change. The progression of this dementia is unpredictable, and in the later stages symptoms are like those of Alzheimer's disease.

The main symptoms of frontotemporal dementia include:

+ decreased inhibition (frequently leading to inappropriate behaviour)

+ apathy and loss of motivation

+ decreased empathy

+ repetitive or compulsive behaviours

+ anxiety and depression.

(Source: https://www.alzheimers.net/)

Diagnosis

A General Practitioner (GP) is usually the first contact when concerns about thinking or memory arise. The GP's role involves identifying symptoms that may indicate dementia, excluding any other possible diagnoses and referring the individual on to specialist services. The GP will also have an ongoing role supporting the individual and their family throughout their illness.

A dementia reference guide for GPs entitled *Dementia: Diagnosis and Management in General Practice* was published by the Irish College of General Practitioners in 2014. This document focuses on key aspects of dementia care including timely diagnosis, early intervention, activation of social supports, multidisciplinary approaches, legal issues and the appropriate use of medication in primary care. While GPs play a key role in the diagnosis of dementia, a confirmatory definitive diagnosis and identification of the dementia sub-type remains a specialist task.

Accurate diagnosis of dementia and identification of the sub-type has become more important for a number of reasons, including the ability to tailor treatments for Alzheimer's disease and vascular dementia, and because of the need to avoid the potentially serious side-effects of antipsychotic drug use in people with Lewy body disease. The earlier the stage of dementia, the more difficult it is to make this diagnosis. The same is true for atypical or complex presentations and cases presenting in people under 65 years of age. Neurologists (doctors who specialise in conditions that affect the brain), geriatricians (doctors who care for older people), old-age psychiatrists and memory clinics (a centre where people are referred if they are diagnosed with dementia) all have a role in dementia diagnosis and sub-typing.

Following a diagnosis, the person with dementia will need considerable emotional and practical support. Local, well-coordinated support services are needed to assist people and their families to cope with the choices and dilemmas confronting them at this often distressing and challenging time.

The Impact of Dementia on the Individual and their Family

The impact of dementia on the quality of life of the older individual and their family can cause fear and anxiety for the older person. To help alleviate these fears it is important that the individual feels supported throughout the progression of their illness. It is also important that the family members and healthcare professionals caring for an older person with dementia also feel supported.

It is accepted that dementia care can be challenging, particularly for family caregivers. However, there is a growing awareness that the older person living with dementia can live well in the community if the necessary supports (statutory, voluntary and community supports) are in place. Better awareness and education around dementia can improve community involvement with dementia care and can mobilise support from the wider community. It gives healthcare professionals, family members and friends a better awareness and appreciation of the situation of the person affected by dementia and it can help to reduce or eliminate fear for all members of the multidisciplinary team who are involved in caring for the person living with dementia.

To help support individuals living with dementia and their families it is important to:

+ create better understanding of dementia through public awareness and health promotion campaigns

+ talk about dementia in order to reduce stigma and raise awareness

+ provide dementia-specific training for all ages, including the person living with dementia

+ provide continuous professional development for carers

+ reduce the isolation of people with dementia

+ advocate for people with dementia who may not be able to self-advocate

+ recognise the rights of people with dementia and of their carers

+ involve people with dementia in their local communities

+ support and educate informal and paid carers, including family carers

+ create and promote peer-led support groups for carers

- improve the quality of care at home and in care homes

- improve dementia training of primary healthcare physicians

- call on governments to create national Alzheimer's disease plans

- increase research into dementia

- create dementia-friendly villages and communities, e.g. Alzheimer's cafés

- create a dementia-friendly journey of care in hospitals from admission to discharge.

Support organisations for the individual and their family

- Alzheimer Society of Ireland (ASI)

- Dementia Services Information and Development Centre (DSIDC)

Dementia-friendly villages/communities

The Alzheimer Society of Ireland (ASI) is leading a Dementia Friendly Communities (DFC) initiative that aims to transform villages, towns, cities and communities into better places for people with dementia to live. There are now seven communities of interest across the country being supported to deliver a range of dementia-friendly activities including community education, volunteering, supporting local businesses to become dementia friendly and improving the social and physical environments.

DFCs seek to encourage more partnerships between non-governmental organisations (NGOs) and local services and to ensure that there is a better awareness, understanding and sensitivity throughout the local community about the needs of people with dementia.

Long-Term Care Options

While current health and social policy is focused on caring for people with dementia in their own homes, there will come a time for many when home care may no longer be feasible or appropriate and long-term residential care is the best option. This can particularly arise when 24-hour care is needed or when the person with dementia is living alone.

It is estimated that 34 per cent of all people with dementia in Ireland live in residential care, a small proportion of whom (1,000 approx.) currently live in specialist care units. The majority of people with dementia currently reside in generic residential care facilities.

It is critical that residential standards for units accommodating people with dementia take appropriate account of the needs of these residents even where the unit in question is not formally described as specialising in dementia. It is also desirable that people with dementia in residential care facilities should be accommodated as close as possible to their home communities.

(Department of Health, 2014.)

CAREGIVER'S 10 COMMANDMENTS

AGREE Never Argue

REDIRECT Never Reason

DISTRACT Never Shame

REASSURE Never Lecture

REMINISCE Never say 'Remember'

REPEAT Never say 'I already told you'

SAY "DO WHAT YOU CAN" Never say 'You can't'

ASK Never Command

ENCOURAGE AND PRAISE Never Condescend

REINFORCE Never Force

(Source: https://dementiaenvironmentaldesign.com)

Case Study: Mr A

Providing Dementia Care

Mr A is a 67-year-old gentleman who lives at home. He has had several falls over the past six months, and it appears he is unable to maintain his safety at home.

Mr A receives support from his local primary healthcare team. He receives regular visits from his public health nurse and home help support. Over the past few visits the home help team have raised some concerns: they have found the front door to Mr A's home open, the heating left on overnight and the kitchen sink taps left on, which has caused damage to the kitchen, meaning Mr A is no longer able to prepare meals for himself.

Mr A also appears disorientated and confused around staff members. He appears to be unsure of the day, date and year. He also appears to be unable to follow simple direction from home help staff.

The public health nurse is notified and requests a GP review. The GP visits Mr A at home: there does not appear to be any underlying infection or any other indicators of an acute exacerbation of his health needs. A cognitive test is performed using a Mini-Mental State Examination Score (MMSE). Mr A's MMSE score is 18/30 which indicates there is an onset of cognitive impairment.

Plan of care

Mr A is admitted to his local nursing home for further assessment and observation, as the GP thinks that Mr X may have early onset dementia.

On admission, Mr A appears incoherent, confused and to have altered communication needs: he appears not to be able to follow verbal instruction or simple commands. Mr A's mobility also appears to be failing: his gait is unsteady, and he requires supervision and the use of a stick to mobilise. Mr A's screening (using MUST) identifies Mr A is at risk of malnutrition.

Task You are tasked with devising a plan of care for Mr A based on his personal profile. Discuss his holistic care needs based on your assessment, referring to Mr A's activities of daily living, i.e. communication, eating and drinking, recreational/social activities, nutrition, elimination, mobility and maintaining a safe environment.

As a healthcare professional, how would you provide effective holistic care for Mr A?

ASSESSMENT TECHNIQUE

As part of your assessment technique for this module you will be required to complete two written assignments as per your assignment brief. Use this case study to help you to plan and write an assignment on an individual living with dementia to whom you will provide care.

chapter 15

PARKINSON'S DISEASE

Parkinson's disease (Parkinson's) is a progressive neurological disorder and is categorised as a movement disorder, as it primarily affects movement. Parkinson's disease will affect people in different ways; the disease will progress more slowly for some people than for others. Parkinson's disease is caused by a loss of a chemical called dopamine. Dopamine is one of the brain's neurotransmitters: it is a chemical that carries information between neurons. Dopamine helps regulate movement, attention, learning and emotional responses. As we age, we all lose some of this chemical, however, it is only when we have lost about 80 per cent of our dopamine that we start to have symptoms.

Parkinson's is the second most common neurodegenerative condition after Alzheimer's. The incidence is 1:500 of the general population, which can be further broken down to 2:100 of the elderly, and 1:10 nursing home residents. It is estimated that there are approximately 9,000 people living with Parkinson's in Ireland.

(Source: https://www.parkinsons.ie)

Signs and Symptoms

Motor symptoms include:

+ tremor (worsened by anxiety)
+ stiffness
+ slowness
+ stooped posture

+ gait disturbance/impaired balance

+ shuffling of feet

+ 'freezing' when walking

+ painful muscle contractions, commonly in the feet.

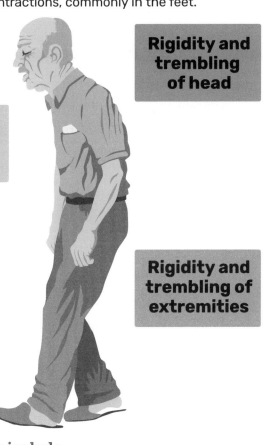

Rigidity and trembling of head

Forward tilt of trunk

Reduced arm swinging

Rigidity and trembling of extremities

Shuffling gait with short steps

Non-motor symptoms include:

+ anxiety

+ bladder and bowel problems

+ depression

+ sensitivity to the heat or cold, for example, excessive sweating

+ fatigue

+ hallucinations

- low blood pressure
- loss of sense of smell
- memory problems
- sleep difficulties.

Treatment for Parkinson's Disease

At present there is no cure for Parkinson's. However, there have been significant improvements in the treatment of the symptoms of Parkinson's in the last twenty years. Treatments include:

- drug therapy
- surgery
- physiotherapy
- speech and language therapy
- occupational therapy.

Research is ongoing into the causes of Parkinson's and into developing new treatments for Parkinson's. As the research methods accelerate, it is likely that there will be better treatments available to improve the quality of life of people with Parkinson's.

Living Well with Parkinson's Disease

Parkinson's disease affects the individual who has been diagnosed with the disease and the person's network of family and friends. Once an individual and their family have had some time to adjust to the diagnosis of Parkinson's disease, it is important that the person realises that they can still live an active life and enjoy a lifestyle that is concurrent with their normal quality of life. It is important that a person is not defined by their disease. Try to empower the individual to keep an optimistic outlook, to continue to enjoy their social and recreational interests and to be willing to adapt and makes changes to facilitate life as the person knows it.

Exercise

Exercise can be especially beneficial for people with Parkinson's in managing symptoms and easing any discomfort associated with movement. It may also improve a person's level of well-being and quality of life. It is also known that physical exercise is essential for maintaining good blood flow to the brain, as well as encouraging production of new brain cells.

The benefits of exercise:

+ maintains flexibility
+ improves balance
+ improves muscle strength
+ improves general functioning
+ improves fitness and stamina
+ provides a sense of achievement and empowerment
+ reduces stress and anxiety.

Prevention

It is important for the individual living with Parkinson's to keep their brain and cognition active and healthy through frequent stimulation. This can also benefit mental and intellectual abilities, which have an impact on brain function. Interestingly, studies have found that engaging in mathematical calculations and brain exercise workouts can help to keep our minds sharp. Puzzles and interactive games can be an effective way of keeping the brain challenged. Participating in brain exercise can defer the onset of dementia and other signs of aging in the brain.

Examples of brain exercise activities include learning something new or returning to education, doing stimulating puzzles such as crosswords and Sudoku and playing interactive games that require you to think such as Scrabble, card games, Monopoly or chess.

Social engagement

It is important that the individual living with Parkinson's continues to socialise with friends and family and remains involved in their local community. This is not only good for the mind, it is also good for the body: it helps the individual to remain active and increases their self-esteem through feeling part of the wider community. It may be useful for some people to consider joining a branch of the Parkinson's Association to meet others who may understand how they feel.

Weight management

Weight can fluctuate for a person living with Parkinson's. Weight loss can occur if there is an increase in movements associated with Parkinson's. These extra movements can present themselves as tremors, which can burn energy. Alternatively, if a person's level of activity decreases because of a change in agility and mobility, it is easy to gain weight. It is useful to seek advice from a dietician in relation to maintaining a healthy, balanced diet and body mass index.

The Impact of Parkinson's on the Individual and their Family

Parkinson's disease can significantly affect an older person's quality of life. The effects of the disease can also impact the individual's family and the wider community. Parkinson's disease can affect many factors associated with positive ageing and the ability of the older person to maintain their independence. Some factors that can be influenced by this degenerative disease include:

+ physical functioning

+ social functioning

+ emotional well-being

+ fears and anxiety

+ stigma

+ loss of autonomy.

To help overcome these factors it can be beneficial for the older person and/or their family to receive the following:

+ education

+ counselling

+ support in relation to everyday care skills and activities of daily living

+ access to medical research

+ membership to support groups

+ advocacy services, including peer advocacy

+ awareness of communication challenges such as hypophonia (soft voice)

+ physical exercise – good for mobility and remaining involved in the community

+ individual assessment and care planning.

It is important that the older person is involved in their care plan and that they agree to support from healthcare professionals, family members and other people who are there to support and assist the person with any element of their care. As Parkinson's disease is a progressive and degenerative disease it is important to review the care plan on a regular basis or as is needed, depending on the individual symptoms displayed.

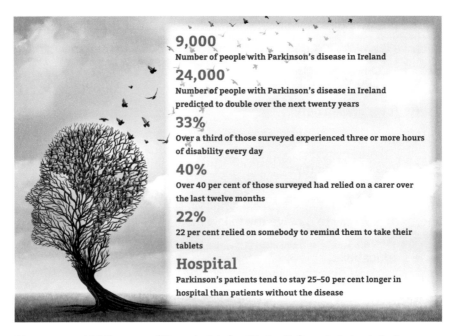

9,000
Number of people with Parkinson's disease in Ireland

24,000
Number of people with Parkinson's disease in Ireland predicted to double over the next twenty years

33%
Over a third of those surveyed experienced three or more hours of disability every day

40%
Over 40 per cent of those surveyed had relied on a carer over the last twelve months

22%
22 per cent relied on somebody to remind them to take their tablets

Hospital
Parkinson's patients tend to stay 25–50 per cent longer in hospital than patients without the disease

(Source: www.irishtimes.com/life-and-style/health-family/how-is-ireland-dealing-with-parkinson-s-disease-1.2609137)

Supportive Therapies and Interventions

There are several therapies that can make living with Parkinson's disease easier and that can help the older person to manage their symptoms from day to day.

Physiotherapy

A physiotherapist can work with the older person, the person's family and as part of the multidisciplinary team (MDT) to help with changes in mobility, muscle stiffness and joint pain through movement (manipulation) and exercise. A physiotherapist will implement an individual care plan for the older person and share this information with the MDT.

Occupational therapy

An occupational therapist (OT) can identify areas of difficulty in the older person's everyday life, for example, their activities of daily living such as dressing, bathing or going to the local shops, and suggest strategies to improve them. The OT can also offer practical advice to the family and to members of the MDT.

Speech and language therapy

About half the people with Parkinson's disease have problems communicating such as slurred speech or poor body language. If an older person has communication difficulties, a speech and language therapist (SLT) can help with these issues to improve speech and use of language.

Medication

Medication can be prescribed by a person's GP or by their consultant if required. Medications are typically prescribed to help reduce some of the signs and symptoms associated with Parkinson's disease, such as a tremor (shaking of the limbs) but will not prevent or cure the degenerative disease.

Surgery: deep brain stimulation

Deep brain stimulation is a surgical technique that is sometimes used to treat Parkinson's disease. A pulse generator (similar to a heart pacemaker) is inserted into the older person's chest wall and a fine wire is placed under the skin and attached to the brain. A tiny electric current is produced from the pulse generator, which runs through the wire and stimulates the part of the brain that is affected by Parkinson's disease. Although surgery does not cure Parkinson's disease, it can ease the symptoms for some people.

(Source: https://www.hse.ie/eng/health/az/p/parkinson's-disease/treating-parkinson's-disease.html)

Parkinson's Association of Ireland

The Parkinson's Association of Ireland is a registered charity that provides support and advice for people living with Parkinson's disease and their family members. It provides a freephone helpline service offering: free, confidential and impartial advice; information and support on a number of subjects, including coping with Parkinson's disease; advice on how to manage expectations; easy-to-understand explanations about Parkinson's disease; and a service that listens without judgment.

Parkinson's is a shared disease; progression to advanced stages is difficult to navigate **for people living with the condition and loved ones/caregivers**

Clinical definitions of Parkinson's over-simplify the full experience; to truly appreciate challenges of living with the condition, the complex physical, mental, social and emotional experience must be included

Physical loss is not always the hardest; people living with Parkinson's also evaluate the condition's impact based on social loss, emotional lows and sometimes cognitive impairment

Dedicated to maintaining a pre-Parkinson's lifestyle, **people living with the condition develop strategies to manage daily activities;** many try to embrace their situation with optimism

Key insights

Parkinson's is not simply a gradual accumulation of symptoms but **a complex transition from a life without Parkinson's to a life as a person living with Parkinson's;** this can vary dramatically (throughout the day and over time) depending on medication/lifestyle

People living with Parkinson's consider themselves **host to an 'unwelcomed guest'**, striving for Parkinson's not to become their identity

People living with Parkinson's become the experts on their version of the condition and rely on a diverse network of experts for support

People living with Parkinson's see the impact on quality of life as central, as **the condition can challenge mood, sleep, daily activities and interpersonal relationships**

(Source: https://parkinsonslife.eu/step-the-lived-experience-of-parkinsons/)

Caring for a Person with Parkinson's Disease

Using Roper, Logan and Tierney's 12 Activities of Daily Living, in caring for a person with Parkinson's disease, we must assist with the following aspects.

1   Maintaining a safe environment

+ Keep the area clutter-free to reduce risk of falls.
+ Keep walking aids within easy reach.

+ Keep call bells within arm's length.

+ Grab rails, ramps and rollators can help a person to mobilise.

2 Communication

+ People who have Parkinson's disease can have problems with the volume of their voice.

+ They can also have problems with speaking too quickly or too slowly: this is known as dysarthria.

+ Encourage the person to speak slowly.

+ Don't try to pretend that you understand if you do not.

+ Handwriting can deteriorate; offer to help with writing letters, notes or postcards if needed.

3 Breathing

In general, a person with Parkinson's disease tends not to have any issues with their breathing. If a person has anxiety or feels stressed this can sometimes exacerbate a person's breathing rate, so be mindful of this possibility and always offer support and reassurance if this happens.

4 Eating and drinking

Dysphagia can occur for a person living with Parkinson's disease. It is important to be mindful of this and to monitor for:

+ coughing or choking episodes during mealtimes

+ wet, gurgled voice during or after meals

+ weight loss, chest infections or dehydration.

Practical tips

+ Try to have mealtimes when medication is working well.

+ Support the person to sit upright.

+ Encourage small mouthfuls.

+ Avoid chatting while the person is eating.

+ Avoid crumbly foods (such as egg, dry toast, biscuits).

+ Offer cold drinks to make swallowing more efficient.

+ Allow the person enough time to eat.

+ Offer assistive aids such as weighted cutlery or a cup with a lid.

If you are concerned about or notice a change in a person's ability to swallow it is important to report this information to the nurse and to other members of the healthcare team. The person will need to be reviewed by a speech and language therapist to ensure that they have a safe swallow and that they are offered a suitable diet consistency.

5   Elimination

Constipation can occur for a person who has Parkinson's disease. A poor diet may be a contributing factor.

Practical tips

+ Encourage a diet with fresh fruit and vegetables.

+ Encourage foods high in fibre.

+ Encourage the person to increase their fluid intake.

Incontinence can be an embarrassing and distressing problem for the person living with Parkinson's. A healthcare professional should always ask: is the problem due to decreased mobility? Or is the person finding it difficult to get to the bathroom on time, as it is located too far away?

Practical tips

+ Try to keep the route to the toilet clear and clutter-free.

+ Keep a urinal or commode, if needed, within easy reach.

+ Is the problem due to difficulty with buttons or zips? Ensure clothing is appropriate, for example, encourage the use of Velcro fasteners or elasticised waist trousers or skirts.

6   Washing and dressing

A person with Parkinson's may require assistance with washing and dressing. It is important to promote the independence of the individual by encouraging them to do as much as they can for themselves.

Be mindful to include the person and offer choice when assisting them with washing and dressing. Remember to always ensure that the privacy and the dignity of the person is protected.

7   Temperature control

One of the non-motor symptoms of Parkinson's is sensitivity to the heat or the cold. An individual may complain about any change in temperature. It is important that you ensure the person is comfortable at all times by reducing heat if a person is too warm or generating heat if they are cold.

Practical tips

✚   Be mindful of environmental temperature changes during winter and summer.

✚   If a person is too warm, open a window, remove clothing, remove bed linen or use a cold compress to help reduce temperature.

✚   If a person is too cold, offer another layer of clothing, offer another blanket, offer the person a hot drink.

8   Mobility

The most common mobility problems are walking, posture and standing from sitting.

Practical tips

✚   **Walking:** give the person enough time, no rushing.

✚   **Posture:** encourage the person to stand up tall and correct their posture regularly.

✦ **Standing from sitting:** ensure the person is sitting in high-backed, firm chairs with arm rests.

9 Work and play

It is important that the individual living with Parkinson's is encouraged to maintain their normal recreational and social activities, as per the person's own interests and hobbies.

10 Sexuality

Some people with Parkinson's can display inappropriate sexual behaviour. This can be related to their medication. It is important that if a person displays any inappropriate sexual behaviour that it is reported to your line manager immediately.

11 Sleep

People with Parkinson's often have trouble with sleep. It is important that a person's sleep pattern is recorded; it may be useful to use a sleep record chart if this is an ongoing issue.

12 Death and dying

Parkinson's disease does not cause death. It can be a contributing factor to pneumonia due to swallowing difficulties, and this can be particularly serious for the older person. It is important that healthcare professionals are aware that a person may have fears and anxieties about death and dying. It can be useful to help relieve these fears by offering advice, support and education in line with your scope of practice. If you feel the person should speak to the nurse or their doctor, it is good practice to report and initiate this request to the MDT so that supports can be implemented.

(Source: https://www.parkinsons.ie/Professionals_ADLs)

INTERESTING FACTS

+ It is estimated that Parkinson's disease affects 9,000 people in Ireland, that is, 1:500 of the general population, which can be further broken down to 2:100 of the elderly and 1:10 nursing home residents.

+ 70 per cent of people with Parkinson's disease will develop a tremor.*

+ Slowness of movement is often described as a difficulty for people with Parkinson's, affecting ability to complete daily tasks at the usual speed and ease, for example, getting dressed or having a shower.

+ This slowness of movement can also affect the way in which the person walks, as it may cause short, shuffling steps.

+ Gentle exercise or physiotherapy can help relax tight muscles and improve mobility.

+ One in five people with Parkinson's disease will develop dementia as they get older.

+ Loss of stability in later stages of Parkinson's disease can lead to falls. It is important that healthcare professionals caring for an individual with a change in mobility outlines care considerations to prevent falls in that person's care plan. Always refer to the nurse and to the care plan for further advice.

*(Source: https://parkinsons.ie/Professionals_What_Is_Parkinsons)

chapter 16

CARDIOVASCULAR DISEASE INCLUDING STROKE

Heart disease (cardiovascular disease) remains the most common cause of death in Ireland. It is currently the cause of one-third of all deaths and one in five premature deaths. Approximately 10,000 people die each year from cardiovascular disease, including coronary heart disease, stroke and other circulatory diseases.

(Source: https://irishheart.ie)

Stroke

A stroke is a serious medical condition that occurs when the blood supply to part of the brain is cut off. Like all organs, the brain needs the oxygen and nutrients provided by blood to function properly. If the supply of blood is restricted or stopped, brain cells begin to die. This can lead to brain damage and possibly death.

In Ireland, strokes are a major health problem. Every year over 8,500 people have a stroke and it is the third largest cause of death, after heart disease and cancer. People who are over 65 years of age are most at risk from strokes.

(Source: https://irishheart.ie)

Risk factors associated with stroke

+ smoking
+ obesity
+ lack of exercise
+ poor diet
+ high blood pressure
+ high cholesterol
+ atrial fibrillation (an irregular heartbeat)
+ diabetes

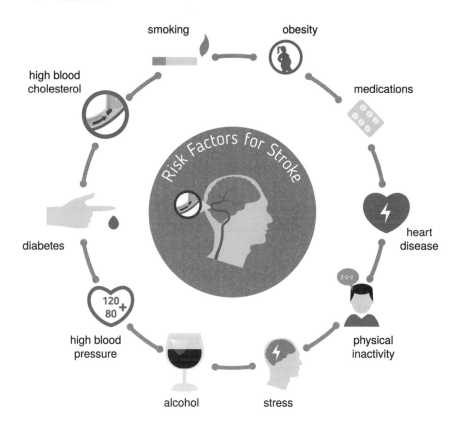

How to recognise if a person is having a stroke

The main stroke symptoms can be remembered with the word **FAST**: Face–Arms–Speech–Time.

+ **Face:** the face may have drooped on one side, the person may not be able to smile, or their mouth or eye may have drooped

+ **Arms:** the person may not be able to lift one or both arms and the arms may remain at their sides because of arm weakness or numbness

+ **Speech:** their speech may be slurred or garbled, or the person may not be able to talk at all despite appearing to be awake

+ **Time:** it is time to dial 112 or 999 immediately if you see any of these signs or symptoms.

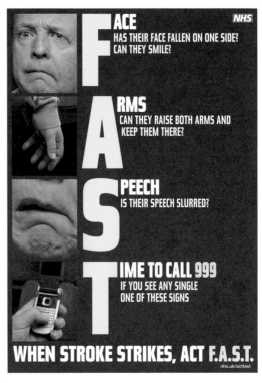

Other signs and symptoms include:

+ numbness or weakness, resulting in complete paralysis of one side of the body

+ sudden loss of vision, or partial loss of vision typically in one eye

+ dizziness and problems with balance and coordination

+ difficulty talking and understanding what others are saying

+ difficulty swallowing

+ sudden and severe headache, unlike any the person has had before, especially if associated with neck stiffness

+ blacking out (in severe cases).

Ischemic strokes

Ischemic strokes occur when blood clots block the flow of blood to the brain. Blood clots typically form in areas where the arteries have narrowed or become blocked by fatty cholesterol-containing deposits known as plaques (this narrowing of the arteries is caused by atherosclerosis). As we get older our arteries become narrower, but certain risk factors can dangerously accelerate the process.

Risk factors include:

+ smoking

+ high blood pressure

+ obesity

+ high cholesterol levels (often caused by a high-fat diet, but can also result from inherited factors)

+ family history of diabetes or heart disease

+ excessive alcohol intake (which can also make obesity and high blood pressure worse, as well as causing heart damage and an irregular heartbeat).

Haemorrhagic strokes

Haemorrhagic strokes (also known as cerebral haemorrhages or intracranial haemorrhages) usually occur when a blood vessel in the brain bursts and bleeds (intracerebral haemorrhage). The main cause of haemorrhagic stroke is high blood pressure (hypertension), which can weaken the arteries in the brain and make them prone to split or rupture.

Risk factors for high blood pressure include:

+ being overweight

+ drinking excessive amounts of alcohol

+ smoking

+ lack of exercise

+ genetic considerations.

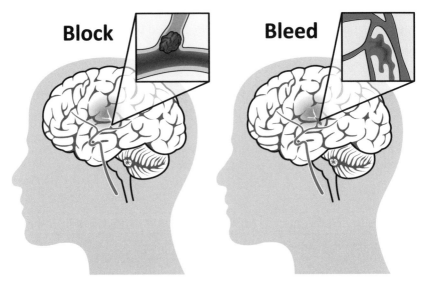

Ischaemic stroke
(embolic and
thrombotic)

Haemorrhagic stroke
(subarachnoid and
intracerebral)

Cognitive impact of a stroke

One or more cognitive functions can be disrupted by a stroke. Cognitive functions include:

+ communication, both verbal and written

+ spatial awareness, i.e. having a natural awareness of where your body is in relation to your immediate environment

+ memory

+ concentration

+ the ability to plan, solve problems and reason about situations
+ the ability to carry out activities of daily living and learned physical activities, such as getting dressed or making a cup of tea.

Stroke rehabilitation

Rehabilitation may include help with:

+ Activities of daily living such as walking, dressing, washing, grooming, cooking, returning to work, driving
+ balance and mobility
+ use of the arm and hand
+ speech and language
+ swallowing safely
+ adapting a healthy diet and lifestyle
+ thinking and understanding
+ memory
+ reading and writing
+ sight
+ well-being and happiness.

The Rehabilitation Team

Physiotherapy

Often, the physiotherapist will provide exercises to improve mobility, balance or use of the affected arm, and will give advice about the best positions for sitting and sleeping.

Occupational therapy (OT)

The OT helps the affected person to become as independent as possible in their daily life, including working, socialising, leisure activities and driving. If the affected person is having a difficulty in any of these areas, the OT will work with them to put together a treatment programme. The OT may also visit the person at home to see what alterations or equipment may be needed to assist them to be as independent as possible.

Speech and language therapy (SLT)

The SLT works on any speech and communication difficulties the person may be having and helps to find the best way for the person to communicate with friends and family. The SLT may also provide exercises to improve speech and use of words and language. The SLT will also advise on any problems swallowing food and drink.

Dysphagia

Dysphagia is the medical term for difficulty swallowing. Difficulties swallowing are common in the first few days after stroke. The affected person may find it hard to eat or drink. A swallow test is one of the first hospital assessments; initially it involves seeing if the person can swallow a little bit of water without choking or coughing. Due to brain damage caused by stroke, eating and drinking may be difficult, as the muscles of chewing and swallowing may be weakened, especially in the early stages of recovery.

Signs and symptoms of dysphagia

+ choking when eating
+ sensation of food getting stuck in the throat or chest, or behind the breastbone
+ coughing or gagging when swallowing
+ drooling or inability to control saliva in the mouth
+ hoarseness
+ unexplained weight loss

+ bringing food back up (regurgitation)

+ difficulty controlling food in the mouth

+ difficulty starting the swallowing process

+ recurrent pneumonia

+ eyes watering when eating

+ 'pooling food' (holding food in the mouth).

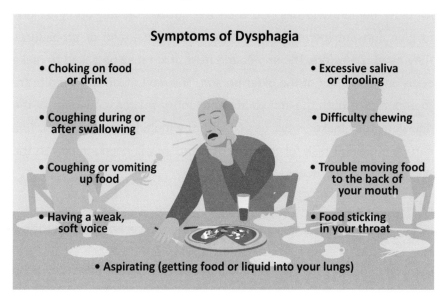

Symptoms of Dysphagia

- Choking on food or drink
- Excessive saliva or drooling
- Coughing during or after swallowing
- Difficulty chewing
- Coughing or vomiting up food
- Trouble moving food to the back of your mouth
- Having a weak, soft voice
- Food sticking in your throat
- Aspirating (getting food or liquid into your lungs)

Dietician

A dietician looks at diet and nutritional requirements. They will monitor what the affected person eats and will advise what food and drinks will suit their needs. They will give the person advice to help them to maintain a healthy lifestyle. If all or part of the person's nutrition requires a feeding tube, the dietician will devise a suitable feeding plan to meet their needs and will monitor progress.

The Impact of a Stroke on the Individual and their Family

A GP may make the initial diagnosis in relation to an older person's stroke and will refer the older person to Accident and Emergency. This can be a frightening experience for the individual and their family members. Most older people who have a stroke and are admitted to hospital will be under the direct care of a doctor, often a geriatrician or possibly a neurologist. An older person who has had a severe stroke may not be conscious to give consent (permission) for the care intervention or procedures they need. Therefore, the immediate next of kin may be asked to make decisions on behalf of the older person. The next of kin will need to try to understand both the immediate and long-term consequences of the decisions they make, in discussion with the multidisciplinary team. This can be a difficult task for the next of kin; they will need support in the decision-making process.

1   Hemiplegia

Hemiplegia means paralysis of half of or one side of a person's body. According to the Irish Heart Foundation, this can occur in about 80 per cent of all people who have had a stroke. The paralysis can be either partial (some loss of sensation) or complete (full loss of sensation): this will depend on the severity of the stroke. The paralysis happens because there is an injury to the part of the brain that transmits messages to the muscles in the arms and legs. As a consequence of the anatomy of the brain, if the right side of the brain is injured, the paralysis affects the left side of the body; if the left side of the brain is injured, the paralysis is on the right side of the body. Balance may also be affected, so the person may be likely to fall or lean sideways in the bed or chair.

(Source: http://irishheart.ie/wp-content/uploads/2017/01/Step_by_Step_ Through_Stroke_-_SEPA_ready.pdf)

If an older person has a weakness to the left side of their body, they may find it difficult to see objects on the left side of their visual field.

2 Difficulties communicating

The two major problems with communication are:

1 not being able to express words

2 not being able to understand the spoken word.

Some people who have had a stroke have difficulty expressing words or may even lose the ability to speak (see the 'Key terms' text box on pp. 139–40), even though they may be able to understand what is being said to them. It is paramount that healthcare professionals do not assume that because the older person is unable to speak that they cannot understand what is being said to them.

3 Loss of intellectual or thinking ability

Loss of intellectual function can affect the older person's ability to pay attention and to concentrate; problem-solving and receiving new information can be overwhelming.

4 Emotional changes

The older person may experience a range of emotional changes and reactions after having a stroke. For example, the person may laugh or cry out for no apparent reason. This is often described as pathological laughter or crying. This can be very distressing for the person and for their carers, but, fortunately, this can usually be helped with medication.

Healthcare professionals including doctors, nurses and health care assistants will assess the older person and will offer support and guidance to the person's family, relatives, friends or carers to help understand and discuss the factors associated with having a stroke.

COMMUNICATION TIPS FOR THE INDIVIDUAL AND THEIR FAMILY

+ Use an array of verbal and non-verbal styles of communication, for example, speech, writing, drawing, gesture and pointing.

+ Allow enough time to respond.

+ Reduce background noise such as television or radio.

+ Repeat important words.

+ Write down important words to clarify meaning (a mini whiteboard can be useful for this).

Role of Relatives and Supports Available

Family, friends and the older person's wider support network can play a crucial role in supporting and encouraging the older person during the different stages of recovery from stroke. The natural response for many carers and relatives is to be protective and to attempt to do too much for the older person: this can limit an older person's ability to maintain their independence, and it can also interfere with opportunities for the older person to practise their skills, including their mobility exercises to help improve their agility.

The role of relatives and carers is to strike a balance between being protective and encouraging independence. It is vital to facilitate the older person to do as much for themselves as they can. It may take longer and require patience, but it is important to a person's independence. This is not only a good practice guideline for family carers, it is also important for healthcare professionals to remember this aspect of care during care interventions.

Stroke support groups for the individual and their circle of support

Stroke support groups can be beneficial to the older person, as they allow the person to meet others and share information regarding similar experiences and their journey of care. Support groups not only provide a meeting place for people affected by stroke, but they also offer an opportunity for an older person's carers to come together. This can also be a very positive aspect of meeting people's social and recreational needs. People in the group can discuss problems and offer advice or support that may have helped them with an issue previously. The groups provide education and information, raise awareness and offer advice on stroke and the ability to live well after a stroke. Some also offer activity programmes and services.

Practical Aspects of Care After Stroke

Eating and drinking

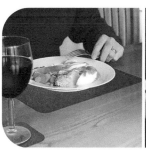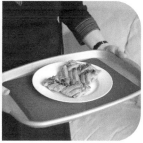

+ Non-slip mats or plates with suction pads are available which stop plates from slipping and make eating with one hand easier.

+ Utensils with thick handles can be easier to use.

+ Meat and other foods should be cut into bite-sized pieces. Cutting up food when the plate is at the table can make the person feel like a child, so if you are assisting a person at mealtimes, cut up the food before the plate is served.

Dressing

When the older person is dressing or if they are being assisted with dressing, ask them to put their affected or weaker arm or leg into their clothes first. Alternatively, when undressing, a person's good arm or leg should be taken out of the clothes first.

Other considerations that can help with washing and dressing are as follows:

+ loose clothing is easier to put on and remove

+ elasticised waistbands mean that no buttons need to be fastened

+ zips are easier to manage than buttons

+ Velcro can be easier to open and close

+ slip-on shoes or a shoehorn assist with footwear

+ sitting at a table with a basin of water on a non-slip mat is easier to manage than trying to wash while standing at a sink

+ electric razors make it easier to shave with one hand

+ special showers are available that allow wheelchair access.

Mobility and transfers

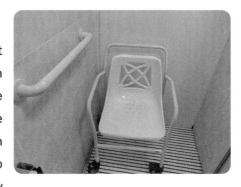

The occupational therapist will advise the older person and their care team on the suitability of beds and chairs. The physiotherapist will advise on the correct transfer technique to the older person independently or with the help of a carer to transfer safely. It is important that family carers and healthcare professionals are aware of 'People Moving and

Handling' techniques in line with best practice guidelines so that the older person is mobilised or transferred safely.

(Irish Heart Foundation, 2017.)

Key terms

Aphasia is a difficulty with language caused when areas of the brain that control language become damaged. Aphasia can affect the ability to talk, read, write or spell, as well as the ability to understand spoken or written language.

Apraxia of speech is an inability to coordinate movement of the tongue muscles because of damage to the brain, even though there is no damage to the muscles needed for the movement.

Aspiration is when food or drink goes into the larynx and enters the airway, causing choking.

Ataxia is a tremor when a person tries to move his or her affected limbs. It may cause the body to become unsteady when standing and walking.

Dysarthria is a motor speech disorder that happens because of weaknesses in or incoordination of the muscles needed to talk, which makes it difficult to pronounce words.

Dysphagia is the medical term for difficulty swallowing (see page 132).

Case Study: Mrs B

Stroke

Mrs B has recently been admitted to a residential care setting (a local nursing home) from hospital following a stroke. She is 78 years old. Mrs B's past medical history includes arthritis of the hands and hip joints, high blood pressure and high cholesterol.

She has lived on her own for the last six years since her husband died. She has two daughters; one is married and lives in England and the other is married and lives in Dublin.

Prior to her stroke, Mrs B was very involved in her local community: she enjoyed going to Mass and attending local GAA games; she volunteered with the local Tidy Towns committee; and she visited her local pub at the weekend. Mrs B had been a smoker, smoking thirty cigarettes a day.

Since the stroke, Mrs B has a left-sided weakness and is unable to walk independently. As per her individualised care plan, she requires the assistance of two people to mobilise in and out of bed with the aid of mechanical aids. Mrs B's skin integrity is fragile as a result of her impaired mobility, and she requires regular re-positioning to promote optimum tissue viability. She has a good cough reflex and no difficulty swallowing but has difficulty at mealtimes. She has some communication difficulties, as her words are slurred and her speech can be incoherent at times, which leads to frustration. Her vision has also been affected by the stroke. Mrs B has a hearing impairment and she wears bi-lateral hearing aids. She suffers from occasional incontinence since her stroke; she can become embarrassed by this and needs full assistance with all her hygiene and personal care needs.

Task

Identify Mrs B's holistic care needs and how you as the healthcare professional would assist Mrs B with these needs.

Pointers to help you to identify Mrs B's holistic care needs:

+ Discuss Mrs B's care needs, i.e. physical, emotional, social, psychological and spiritual impact needs.

+ Discuss how these needs can be met.

+ Identify required care equipment and other aids.

+ Discuss how to prevent Mrs B from getting pressure sores.

+ Discuss procedures relating to the safety and security of Mrs B in terms of meeting her needs.

+ Discuss the importance of safe and hygienic work practices.

+ Identify two key points that will contribute to enhanced quality of life for Mrs B.

+ Identify reporting procedures for changes in Mrs B's well-being and identify relevant records that must be maintained during her care.

+ Make recommendations regarding the care of Mrs B.

chapter 17

MENTAL ILLNESS

There is an assumption that developing mental health problems is a normal part of ageing, but this is not the case. It is important to remember that most people remain in good mental health throughout their lives and live well into their advancing years. However, the most common mental health issues that the elderly can develop are depression and anxiety.

Depression

Depression describes a range of moods, from feeling sad, hopeless and disinterested to being unable to cope with and participate in everyday life and daily living. This feeling can prevail and remain for weeks or perhaps months.

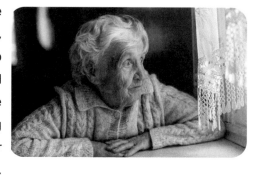

Depression can affect anyone, of any culture, age or background. However, research indicates that more older people are affected than any other age group. This is because the ageing population is much more vulnerable to factors that can cause depression, such as:

+ being widowed or divorced

+ being retired or unemployed

+ physical disability or illness

+ loneliness and isolation.

Signs and symptoms of depression

- ✚ Feelings of hopelessness
- ✚ Feelings of sadness, low mood and tearfulness
- ✚ Loss of interest in daily activities
- ✚ Loss of interest in personal hygiene or personal appearance
- ✚ Difficulties concentrating
- ✚ Alteration in sleep pattern
- ✚ Loss of interest in eating and drinking
- ✚ Loss of interest in or avoidance of social interaction
- ✚ Withdrawal from normal social or recreational activities.

If a person experiences these signs and symptoms they should always be taken seriously. A healthcare professional caring for the older person may be the first person to notice a change in mood. Any change in mood or behaviour should be reported to the line manager and information shared with the multidisciplinary team. There is a range of supports available for the older person who may be experiencing depression, such as psychological supports and medical treatments.

Anxiety

We live in a fast-paced world. This can cause many people, including the older person, to experience nervousness, stress or worry at different times. This is a normal response to a stressful experience or potential threat to our well-being or our quality of life. If an older person appears to be unable to deal with worry or a stressful situation, they may experience anxiety. Anxiety is when feelings of nervousness, stress or worry become more intense, ranging from continual worry to fear and panic. The challenges and vulnerabilities associated with ageing have the potential to cause anxiety in later years.

Signs and symptoms of anxiety

✚ disturbed sleep

✚ tense muscles

✚ morbid thoughts

✚ irritability

✚ fear of the worst-case scenario always occurring

✚ anxiety attacks.

Depression   ## Anxiety

Frustration

Sadness

Restlessness

Trembling

Feeling worthless

Irritability

Trouble thinking, concentrating or making decisions

Increased breathing rate

Feeling nervous or powerless

Loss of interest in normal activities

Excessive worrying

Thoughts of suicide or death

Unexplained physical ailments, such as headaches or stomach aches

Having a sense of impending danger or panic

Tiredness

Agitation

High heart rate

Disturbance in sleep or appetite

Sweating

---

12 STEPS TO GOOD MENTAL HEALTH

1 Keep physically active.

2 Eat well, with nutritionally balanced meals and correct portion size.

3 Drink alcohol in moderation or not at all.

4 Value and care for yourself and others.

5 Keep in touch with friends and loved ones.

6 Get involved and make a contribution.

7 Learn new skills.

8 Do something creative.

9 Get in touch with your spiritual side.

10 Get in touch with nature.

11 Talk about your feelings.

12 Look for help.

(Source: https://www2.hse.ie/conditions/mental-health/clinical-depression/
clinical-depression-diagnosis.html, HSE, 2019.)

Supports

Alzheimer Society of Ireland

Helpline: 1800 341 341

www.alzheimer.ie

Aware

helping to defeat depression

Helpline: 1800 80 48 48 (7 days, 10.00 a.m. to 10.00 p.m.)

www.aware.ie

Samaritans

befriending service supporting those passing through personal crises

24 Hour Helpline: 116 123

www.samaritans.ie

Seniorline

confidential listening service for older people by older people

Helpline: 1800 80 45 91

www.thirdageireland.ie

Active Retirement Ireland

01 873 3836

www.activeirl.ie

Age Action Ireland

01 873 3836

www.ageaction.ie

Age and Opportunity

01 805 7709

www.ageandopportunity.ie

Family Carers Ireland

1800 240 724

www.familycarers.ie

Friends of the Elderly

01 873 1855

www.friendsoftheelderly.ie

Mental Health Ireland

01 284 1166

www.mentalhealthireland.ie

SECTION 4

PERSON-CENTRED END-OF-LIFE CARE

IN THIS SECTION YOU WILL LEARN ABOUT:

+ Person-centred end-of-life care for the older person

+ How to recognise if a person's condition is deteriorating

+ The skills and competencies needed to provide dignity and respect to the older person receiving end-of-life care

+ The role of the HCA in in providing end-of-life care as a member of the multidisciplinary team

+ The role of the HCA in assisting the individual with end-of-life care once death has occurred

chapter 18

PERSON-CENTRED END-OF-LIFE CARE

End-of-Life Care

The provision of end-of-life care can carry with it an array of emotions for all healthcare professionals, but particularly for a student health care assistant. In addition to fear, anxiety and uncertainty, a student health care assistant may feel ill-equipped, as a learner, to deliver such care. It is important that student health care assistants are supported in all aspects of clinical practice in their clinical area when providing end-of-life care to an older person. It is just as important to use this supported time as a learner to shadow health care assistants and nurses when they are providing such care.

Furthermore, it is one of the roles of the health care assistant to be involved in the delivery of end-of-life care. It is important that student health care assistants have an awareness of end-of-life care and that they learn about this type of care. In saying that, it is normal to feel overwhelmed when exposed to the delivery of end-of-life care. Ultimately, it is important that this care skill is approached with dignity, respect and professionalism.

Providing such care may not necessarily get easier the more you are exposed to death and dying, but your care skills and your confidence in the provision of end-of-life care will improve with experience. It is important to remember that person-centred care is a key component of end-of-life care: each person you care for will have individual fears, anxieties, wishes and beliefs that need to be respected as the person approaches an active end-of-life stage.

End-of-life care can be from the point of receiving a life-limiting diagnosis through the months before death, up to and including the final hours: it is a continuum rather than a point in time. We can use the term 'end-of-life care' to refer to the care of people with advanced life-limiting conditions, for whom death within one to two years is likely, as well as those in the terminal phase of illness. It also encompasses care of the bodily remains of the deceased person.

(Source: https://hospicefoundation.ie/aboutus/hospice-palliative-and-end-of-life-care/definitions)

At the end of life, each story is different, and each older person will have individual end-of-life care needs. It is important to identify these needs and to accept that healthcare professionals have a duty to provide holistic end-of-life care that is considerate of the individual needs of the older person and of their cultural beliefs and preferences.

End-of-life symbol

✚ This symbol appears on many of the resources developed by the Hospice Friendly Hospitals Programme to respectfully identify items connected with the end-of-life stage in hospitals and residential care settings.

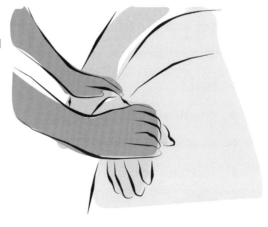

✚ In conjunction with good practice in care facilities, the symbol aims to add respect and solemnity to items used following the death of a person and to make resources relating to the end of life instantly identifiable.

✚ The symbol is inspired by ancient Irish history and is not associated with any one religion or denomination. The three-stranded white spiral represents the interconnected cycle of life – birth, life and death. The white outer circle represents continuity, infinity and completion. Purple was chosen as the background colour as it is associated with nobility, solemnity and spirituality.

Who is involved in providing end-of-life care?

Healthcare professionals act as advocates for patients, residents or service users; we provide a voice for the residents we care for. It is important to remember that we can initiate a palliative care referral with the resident's GP as the resident's needs arise or change, which we will ascertain by monitoring and reporting any distressing symptoms associated with life-limiting illness. The following is a non-exhaustive list of these symptoms:

✚ pain

✚ pressure sores

✚ swallowing difficulties

✚ shortness of breath

✚ fatigue

✚ anxiety

✚ depression

+ constipation

+ reduced appetite

+ nausea

+ vomiting.

Key Points to Remember

+ End-of-life care involves the process of assessing, monitoring and providing physical, emotional and social care needs to a person and their family at the end of their life.

+ End-of-life care is a continuum of care.

+ End-of-life care needs differ for each individual.

+ It is appropriate to talk about end-of-life care needs with the individual but remember it must be done with compassion and empathy.

How to Recognise if a Person's Condition is Deteriorating

A person may:

+ withdraw from social activities

+ spend more time in bed, remaining bed-bound for over 50 per cent of the time

+ have increased sleep requirements

+ express a realisation that they are dying

+ have an inability to heal/recover; residents may have poor tissue viability or may develop pressure areas

+ have increased swelling in their limbs or body

- have a decrease in their oral intake

- have deterioration in their functional ability, for example, their mobility may decline

- be more susceptible to frequent or reoccurring infections

- have weight loss (more than 10 per cent of body weight in the last six months/BMI below 18)

- display a general physical decline, becoming more dependent with activities of daily living

- have multiple diseases impacting on their well-being

- have an increased frequency of admissions to acute care

- lose the ability to communicate in a meaningful way

- have difficulty swallowing and very poor nutritional intake

- be incontinent of bowel and bladder

- be unable to change position, sit unsupported, hold head up or smile

- have episodes of fever and infection

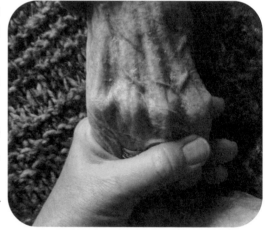

- be at high risk of pressure injury, hip fracture, pneumonia and urinary tract infection, all of which are associated with risk of death within six months.

Pain Management

+ The word 'pain' comes from the Latin *poena,* meaning a fine, a penalty.

+ Pain is a unique experience and how people perceive pain is a vital determinant in how they experience pain. This will influence the pain severity and longevity.

+ Pain and pain threshold can be referred to as being a subjective experience.

+ The International Association for the Study of Pain describes pain as 'an unpleasant sensory and emotional response associated with actual or potential tissue damage or describes in terms of such damage'.

(Source: https://www.iasp-pain.org)

The healthcare professional's goal of care

1. Acknowledge the resident's pain: ask them about their pain and use skills of observation.

2. Assess, then aim to eliminate, reduce and relieve the pain experience. Use the Numerical Pain Scale or the Abbey Pain Score (see p. 157; see Appendix 6).

3. Support the resident and enhance their coping mechanisms to support their pain needs. Be mindful that it is only the registered nurse who can administer pharmacological intervention; however, health care assistants can provide non-pharmacological interventions to relieve pain.

Task Working in groups, list and discuss what non-pharmacological interventions you can use to help relieve pain or discomfort for a person you are caring for.

> **Pain is whatever the experiencing person says it is, existing whenever the experiencing person says it does.**
>
> (Source: Clarke, K.A., Iphofen, R., 2008.)

Psychological symptoms of pain

As well as physical symptoms of pain and discomfort, a person can also experience psychological symptoms of pain:

+ reliving previous experiences of pain

+ anxiety regarding the underlying meaning of the pain

+ feelings of hopelessness

+ feelings of frustration

+ fear that the pain will not be relieved

+ anger at healthcare professionals for not relieving pain

+ fear of being ill

+ fear of dying or not getting better.

Pain Management: LIVE

L   **Locate**

I   **Intensity**

V   **Validate** feelings of pain

E   **Evaluate** care given

(Source: hseland.ie)

Pain assessments

The Numerical Pain Scale

+ Pain is rated from 0 to 10.

+ Residents are asked to rate their pain from 0 to 10, with 0 being the least pain and 10 being the worst pain.

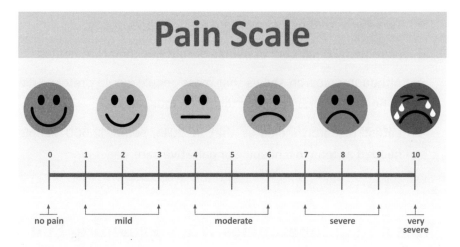

The Abbey Pain Score

+ Used to assess pain for residents with communication difficulties.

+ Assessment of pain for residents with dementia and other communication difficulties is assessed in six areas:

  1 Vocalisation

  2 Facial expression

  3 Change in body language

  4 Behavioural changes

  5 Physiological changes

  6 Physical change

Key Facts on Death, Dying and Bereavement in Ireland

+ An average of 28,000 deaths occur in Ireland each year.

+ On average, eighty people die in Ireland each day.

+ Some ten people are directly affected by each death.

+ Two-thirds of those who die are over 65 years of age.

+ More than 70 per cent of people die outside their own homes.

+ Although research shows that most people would prefer to die at home, this only happens for one in four people.

+ Latest research indicates that in 2016, some 12,500 people needed access to a hospice or palliative care.

(Source: https://hospicefoundation.ie/supporting/wayswesupport/key-facts)

Skills and Competencies When Providing End-of-Life Care

Palliative care

+ A palliative care approach is focused on improving the quality of life of individuals and their families.

+ It is provided in all healthcare settings.

+ It involves providing holistic care to the individual and their family members/loved ones.

+ The palliative approach is not delayed until the end stages of an illness.

+ There is earlier intervention to initiate comfort-focused care to reduce pain and suffering.

+ Palliative care also promotes understanding of loss and bereavement.

Palliative care focuses on promoting comfort through relieving pain and other symptoms. The aim of palliative care is to enhance the quality of life of individuals living with life-limiting conditions whilst providing care and supporting their families. Palliative care uses a team approach to address the needs of residents and their families. The team comprises doctors, nurses, carers and other specialists who work with the resident and their family throughout the person's end-of-life journey.

Members of the healthcare team must be respectful of the older person's individual care plan when providing end-of-life care. It is useful to be mindful of the following points:

+ the person's values, concerns, fears and personal goals for care

+ the person's wishes and choices regarding end-of-life care

+ the person's understanding of their illness and prognosis

+ the person's physical, social, emotional, spiritual and cultural needs

+ the person's preferred place of care and death including the option of a single room or returning home – depending on services available to support this

+ what to do if there is a change in the person's condition, which should include decisions regarding when a resident should or should not be transferred to an acute hospital

+ interventions that may be considered or undertaken in an emergency, such as antibiotics and cardiopulmonary resuscitation (CPR)

+ any other matter that the resident considers important.

Reflection

The focus of care should be 'living life to the end'.

As a healthcare professional, how can you help an older person to live life to the end?

How can you promote the older person's quality of life?

Role of the HCA in Assisting the Nurse with Provision of End-of-Life Care

HIQA outlines the role of all healthcare professionals, including health care assistants, in their national standards for the care of the older person. The standards identify that all healthcare professionals, when providing end-of-life care, should ensure that:

+ residents receive palliative care that supports and respects their dignity

+ each resident receives palliative care based on their assessed needs

+ each resident continues to receive care at the end of their life which respects their dignity and autonomy.

(HIQA, 2016.)

Other key considerations

+ Ensure care plans are in place to meet the end-of-life needs of the person and their families.

+ The person's needs should be communicated and coordinated clearly within the residential centre and other healthcare settings.

+ Healthcare professionals and non-clinical staff should possess an appropriate level of knowledge, skills, competence and confidence to care for residents approaching the end of life.

Healthcare professionals should also be mindful of the following:

+ Everyone has the right to be cared for and to die with dignity and respect.

+ Everyone deserves to have access to the best-quality care at the end of life.

+ People facing death and bereavement have the right to be listened to, and their wishes respected.

+ Ireland's healthcare system has a responsibility to provide best-quality palliative care nationwide.

As healthcare professionals, we only get one chance to care for someone at the end of their lives. We want to ensure that we get this right. We want each person we care for to have a dignified death and for their wishes and beliefs to be respected. In my experience, when I have asked a person about their end-of-life care preferences most people speak about being surrounded by loved ones, having privacy, having their favourite music playing in the background and being free from pain.

Changes That May Be Observed When a Person Enters an Active End-of-Life Stage

It is first important to identify some of the changes that healthcare professionals may observe when a person is entering an active end-of-life stage:

+ As a person's end-of-life journey progresses beyond the early stage, there may be a change in the presentation of how the person presents physically.

+ The person may become bedbound.

+ The person may have altered consciousness or may be unconscious.

✦ The person may take little or no food or fluid.

✦ The person may be unable to swallow oral medications.

✦ The person may be peripherally cyanosed and/or cold. Peripherally cyanosed means that a person's colour will change due to poor circulation, which can be first seen as blue/purple tinge to the peripheries (fingers and toes) and then more centrally (to the rest of the body, the trunk and limbs).

✦ The person may have altered breathing patterns. Cheyne–Stokes respiration is an abnormal pattern of breathing characterised by progressively deeper and sometimes faster breathing, followed by a gradual decrease that results in a temporary stop in breathing called an apnoea.

✦ One may hear an audible respiratory rattle, or the person may have an increase in secretions.

✦ Monitor the person for any signs of constipation and discomfort. The following all increase the risk of constipation: a reduced dietary intake; an inability to take laxatives; the body systems shutting down; and the use of analgesia/opioids.

✦ The person may be incontinent: the body's muscles relax, and the body's contents may be emptied.

✦ The person may become confused, restless and/or possibly appear agitated. This may be caused by a reduction in oxygen to the brain, metabolic changes, dehydration and the use of some opioid/pain medications.

✦ The person's ability to swallow food/fluids/oral medications diminishes significantly. The person may now be unable to tolerate any foods/fluids/oral medications due to risk of aspiration. A person may become NPO: *Nil per os*, Latin for 'nothing by mouth', a medical instruction to withhold oral intake of food and fluids.

It is important to remember that every person's end-of-life journey is unique. Not all symptoms may be present for each individual. A person may present with one or more of the outlined signs and symptoms or none at all. Some people can take their last breath without ever having any of the signs and symptoms that we associate with the continuum of end-of-life care.

+ Remember: even when a person appears to have altered consciousness, they may still be able to hear our voices.

+ It is imperative to be sensitive, gentle and to use a reassuring touch.

+ Knock on the person's door before entering, respect their privacy and dignity, identify yourself, tell the person your name and why you are there (for example, to reposition them, to ensure they are comfortable, to perform oral care, to administer a medication, to sit and hold their hand).

+ Be aware of the need for a quiet environment and soft lighting. Consider the use of music liked by the resident.

+ Family members can be encouraged to replace professionals in the 'inner circle' of care if they wish. Teaching the family member simple skills such as hand massage and basic oral/mouth care, if permitted by local policy, will encourage a sense of purpose and intimacy (HIQA).

+ Ideally, residents would have a single room.

+ Ideally, there would be a family room or quiet area made available to a resident's family members.

+ Comfortable seating/sleeping facilities are helpful.

+ Offering family members tea and sandwiches can be a comfort.

+ Sometimes just being there, being a presence, saying nothing can be comforting; remember that 'silence is golden'.

✚ Try and allow some time for staff to possibly sit with the resident and their family members.

✚ Ensure general tidiness of the room.

✚ Involve the family: communicate any care interventions you may be performing and ask them if they have any special requests or wishes.

✚ A comfort basket for the resident's family is a nice idea, containing, for example, items such as toiletries, towels or tissues.

End-of-Life Care Once Death Has Occurred

Caring for the remains of a deceased person is one part of the overall continuum of care given to people at the end of life and those close to them. At all times the dignity and respect of the deceased person must be maintained.

Before the removal of the deceased by the funeral directors, local procedures should be in place and followed to ensure that staff members care for the remains of the person who has died in a culturally sensitive, dignified and safe manner.

The needs of family members should be sought and met. Family members should be contacted if not already present. They should be offered sympathy and support, and any queries they may have should be clarified. It is important that as a health care assistant you make yourself aware of local policies that are in place in relation to end-of-life care.

Case Study: Mr C

Background

My husband went to the doctor (our local GP) in November complaining about not being able to keep food down, nausea, lethargy and abdominal cramps. The GP did a series of tests (blood tests and a physical examination). It was clear that my husband needed to be referred to an acute setting for further tests. A series of diagnostics tests were performed in our local hospital and when the results came back, they diagnosed my husband with cancer of the liver, stomach and pancreas.

We were told he had two to six months to live. After he was diagnosed, the doctors and other members of the multidisciplinary team were very supportive to my husband and me. We had no idea this was coming; neither of us were prepared for it. We were numb. I found it hard to accept it. I remember crying. As well as trying to come to terms with the diagnosis, we were very concerned that my husband would suffer and experience pain. We were assured and supported by the nurses and health care assistants that my husband would receive great care and that they would help to monitor him for any signs of pain or discomfort. My husband was then referred to the specialist palliative care team.

Context

Mr C is a 75-year-old former hospital chaplain who was well until he developed nausea and vomiting, abdominal cramps and general malaise.

Mr C now requires more assistance with his activities of daily living (grooming, dressing, hygiene needs, personal care needs, toileting needs, mobility, eating and drinking, social inclusion and psychological support needs). Mr C's wife is no longer able to care for her husband at home. Mr C appears to have an increased somnolence and is withdrawn from his network of family and friends. Mr C also has worsening symptoms and pain. Mr C and his wife spoke to their local GP and palliative care team about additional supports. It was decided that Mr C required full nursing care; all parties agreed that the best place to care for Mr C would be in his local community hospital where he would have 24-hour care support. Mr C is currently receiving palliative care within his local community hospital. Mr C's wife is finding the transition hard. She cries during visits and says to staff, 'How long is left? I hate to see him like this.'

On entering Mr C's bedroom you feel he has deteriorated: his colour has changed (his lips, fingers and toes appear cold to touch), you hear him moaning, his lips are dry, his heels are red and tender, his eyes are sunk and he does not respond to your voice.

Task

As the health care assistant providing care to Mr C today, describe how you would provide palliative care to Mr C and offer support to Mr C's wife and family.

Group discussion

+ What are your roles and responsibilities for caring for Mr C, his wife and extended family members over the next number of days, weeks or months?

+ How can you provide holistic care comfort to Mr C in the last days of his life?

+ What physical, emotional, psychological, social and other care can you provide at this time?

SECTION 5

CARE SERVICES, SAFEGUARDING AND POSITIVE OPTIONS

IN THIS SECTION YOU WILL LEARN ABOUT:

+ Preparing and planning for retirement

+ Voluntary and statutory care

+ Health Service Executive

+ Nursing home care

+ Home care supports

+ Health Information Quality Authority (HIQA) and its standards

+ The importance of safeguarding the vulnerable person at risk of abuse

+ Positive leisure, retirement and lifelong learning opportunities for the older person

+ The impact of moving from home to a nursing home

+ Challenges faced by the older person in relation to adapting to a new environment

+ The role of the All Ireland Gerontological Nurses Association (AIGNA)

+ The role of members of the multidisciplinary team, including the speech and language therapist, occupational therapist and physiotherapist, in providing care to the older person

chapter 19

SUPPORT AGENCIES FOR THE OLDER PERSON

Task Working in groups, list some voluntary and statutory services that are available to the older person. Then, research one voluntary and statutory organisation in detail.

Statutory Agencies

Statutory agencies are public sector bodies that are tasked with performing specific functions on behalf of the government. They are funded by the government through an allocation of money from the Department of Health. These agencies can be regulatory bodies or advisory bodies. Regulatory bodies are regulated by the law, for example, the Health Information Quality Authority (HIQA). Advisory bodies provide advice in line with evidence-based practice, for example, the Pre-Hospital Emergency Care Council (PHECC).

The Health Service Executive (HSE)

The HSE was established in 2005 under the Health Act 2004. It is responsible for acute hospitals, mental health services, social care, primary care, health and well-being, the national ambulance service and community healthcare services.

Support services are available from a variety of different agencies including the Department of Health, the Department of Social Protection, local authorities and voluntary organisations. The HSE's mission is to ensure that people in Ireland are supported by quality health and social care services and can avail of safe, compassionate and high-quality care.

The following is a non-exhaustive list of agencies and websites supported by the HSE.

Statutory agencies	<ul><li>Irish Blood Transfusion Service</li><li>Food Safety Authority of Ireland</li><li>Health and Social Care Professionals Council (CORU)</li><li>Health Information and Quality Authority</li><li>Health Products Regulatory Authority</li><li>Health Research Board</li><li>Irish Medical Council</li><li>Irish Mental Health Commission</li><li>National Cancer Registry Ireland</li><li>Nursing and Midwifery Board of Ireland</li><li>Pre-Hospital Emergency Care Council</li></ul>
Health agencies	<ul><li>General Practitioner (GP)</li><li>Community and residential care services</li><li>Health Protection Surveillance Centre</li><li>Local authority departments</li><li>Paramedics</li></ul>

Health agencies *contd.*	+ Ambulance services
	+ Chemists
	+ Opticians
	+ Chiropodists
	+ Physiotherapists
	+ Dentists
	+ Home help
	+ Public Health Nurse
	+ Day centres
	+ Social workers
	+ Speech and language therapists
Health promotion initiatives	+ GetIrelandActive.ie
	+ Quit.ie

The Health Information Quality Authority (HIQA)

HIQA is an independent authority that exists to improve the health and social care services for the people of Ireland. National quality standards are enforced in both public and private nursing homes by HIQA and their inspection reports are available online and can be accessed via their website (www.HIQA.ie).

HIQA's standards team sets national standards for health and social care services to:

+ provide a common language to identify what high-quality, safe, person-centred care looks like

+ create a platform for services to improve the quality and safety of the care they deliver by identifying strengths and highlighting opportunities for improvement

✚ help and support people using services to understand what they should expect from a service

✚ promote evidence based upon practice that is up to date, effective and consistent.

HIQA Current National Standards

The current national standards that apply to the provision of care for the older person in residential care in Ireland are detailed in the HIQA document, 'National Standards for Residential Care Settings for Older People in Ireland' (HIQA, 3 May 2016). These standards are available to download from www.hiqa.ie.

The standards are grouped into eight key themes:

1   **Person-centred care and support**

This standard relates to how the nursing home places residents at the centre of the nursing home's service. This includes providing person-centred care services and protecting residents' rights.

2   **Effective services**

This standard relates to how nursing homes deliver optimal outcomes for residents using best available evidence and information.

3   **Safe services**

This standard relates to how nursing homes protect residents through preventing and minimising the risk of harm and learning from instances of things going wrong.

4   **Health and well-being**

This standard relates to how nursing homes identify and promote the best health outcomes and well-being for each resident, and how the nursing home develops the ongoing improvement of health and well-being for residents.

5   **Leadership, governance and management**

This standard identifies the arrangements put in place by the nursing home for accountability in decision-making, risk management and in meeting its strategic, legal and financial obligations.

6   **Use of resources**

This standard looks at using resources effectively and efficiently to deliver best achievable outcomes for the money and resources used.

7   **Responsive workforce**

This standard identifies the planning, recruitment, managing and organising of staff with the necessary numbers, skills and abilities to respond to the needs of residents.

8   **Use of information**

This standard actively identifies the importance of using information as a resource for planning, delivering, monitoring, managing and improving services.

(HIQA, 2016.)

HIQA is also responsible for:

+ monitoring and inspecting services
+ providing guidance on health information
+ carrying out health technology assessments.

HIQA's Inspection Services

HIQA's Older People's inspection team are legally responsible for the monitoring, inspection and registration of care settings for older people (such as nursing homes) in Ireland.

During inspections the HIQA team aims to meet as many people as possible who are involved in the provision of holistic care to the service user, including residents and family members. HIQA may also wish to speak with members of the multidisciplinary team including staff nurses, health care assistants and the person in charge. HIQA like to meet those involved in the everyday provision of care in order to gather an insight into the daily running of the nursing home and the effectiveness of care provided within each individual setting.

HIQA use regulations and national standards to monitor and inspect care settings providing care to the older person in Ireland. HIQA carry out announced, unannounced and thematic inspections. Over the last number of years, HIQA have carried out thematic inspections in the area of Dementia and Restrictive Practice (the use of restraints, for example, physical restraints, the use of bed rails, environmental restraints, not allowing a person access to a specific part of their environment by denying access to a walking aid/frame).

During these HIQA inspections, the inspectors seek to know that older people who are receiving residential care:

+ are safe

+ have their rights respected

+ are included in decisions about their care

+ are provided with holistic, person-centred care

+ are enjoying a good quality of life (HIQA, 2019).

After each individual inspection, HIQA publish a report into the findings of their inspections. This report identifies if the care setting is compliant or non-compliant with HIQA standards. The report may also include an action plan if there are improvements to be made following the inspection's findings. These reports are published on the HIQA website and can be a useful resource for an older person and their family members seeking to gather information about a specific care setting.

Voluntary Agencies

Voluntary support agencies are run by a group of individuals who share a common goal or agreement. They are usually run by volunteers, and typically depend on funding from fundraising or donations. Voluntary agencies can also be supported by registered charitable agencies and through public funding.

Age Action Ireland

Age Action Ireland is an independent national development agency for older people. It provides a network of support systems for older people, and it also advocates and campaigns for older people and their carers. It promotes better policies and services for older people in an ageing population. (www.ageaction.ie)

Age & Opportunity

Age & Opportunity is a national organisation that provides a range of opportunities for older people who want to get more involved 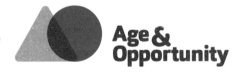 in arts and culture, sport and physical activity, civic engagement and personal development.(www.ageandopportunity.ie)

Alone

ALONE is an independent charity that works with the 1 in 5 older people who are homeless, socially isolated, living in deprivation or in crisis. (www.alone.ie)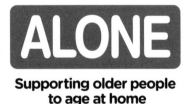

Active Retirement Ireland (ARI)

ARI is a national network of local active retirement associations whose aim is to enable retired people to enjoy full and active lives. ARI also advocates for older people. (www.activeirl.ie)

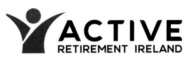

Irish Senior Citizens Parliament

The Irish Senior Citizens Parliament represents the interests of senior citizens and promotes their views to government on issues affecting older people such as income, health or housing. (www.iscp.wordpress. com)

Retirement Planning Council of Ireland

The Retirement Planning Council of Ireland aims to help people to prepare for the period of their lives that begins after they retire from work and to assist them with that transition. (www.rpc.ie)

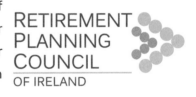

(Source: https://www.hse.ie/eng/services/list/3/ carerssupport/caringforolderpeople.html)

Other services to consider when caring for older people

+ Day services

+ Meals on Wheels

+ Family Carers Ireland

+ Care Alliance Ireland

+ Older Women's Network

+ Acquired Brain Injury Ireland

+ Alzheimer's Association of Ireland

+ Arthritis Ireland

+ Chronic Pain Ireland.

Services that Support Caring for Older People

Home Support Services

The HSE Home Support Service (formerly called the Home Help Service or Home Care Package Scheme) aims to help and support older people to remain in their own homes for as long as possible and to support carers to help care for the older person in their own homes, by offering supportive assistance with activities of daily living for the older person.

The Nursing Homes Support Scheme

The Nursing Homes Support Scheme (also known as the 'Fair Deal' scheme) is a scheme of financial support for people who need long-term nursing-home care. Under the Nursing Homes Support Scheme, an older person will make a contribution towards the cost of their care and the State will pay the balance. This applies whether the nursing home is public, private or voluntary. For an older person to be eligible to apply for the scheme, the person must be living ordinarily in the State for at least a year.

A Care Needs Assessment will be carried out by a nurse or another appropriate healthcare professional. The assessment will include identification of the level of support required for the older person to perform their activities of daily living. A decision is then made based on the Care Needs Assessment as to whether or not the older person will require long-term care in a nursing home or community long-term care setting.

(Health Service Executive, 2018.)

Each care setting will discuss the cost of the nursing home with the older person and their family members during the preliminary stages of seeking information about the care home.

There are a number of Nursing Homes Support Offices located in different regions throughout the country that can offer the older person and their family members advice and support in relation to finding the most suitable long-term care setting to meet their individual needs, choices and preferences.

chapter 20

SAFEGUARDING THE VULNERABLE OLDER PERSON

The Importance of Safeguarding the Vulnerable Person at Risk of Abuse

In December 2014, the HSE launched a new national policy referred to as 'Safeguarding Vulnerable Persons at Risk of Abuse'. This policy replaced existing policies in relation to the detection and reporting of abuse and elder abuse in Ireland's health and social care services.

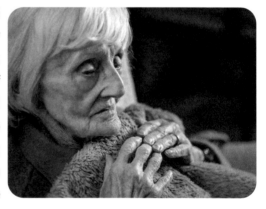

It is paramount that healthcare professionals have an awareness and understanding of this policy, which is fundamental to providing a high-quality, safe service. It is essential to your role as a healthcare worker to understand what abuse is and the steps to take if a concern is made known to you.

It is important to be aware that local policies and procedures exist depending on where you are working: each care setting will have developed a co-existing safeguarding policy within their own set of policies and procedures. It is vital that, as a healthcare professional, you make yourself aware of the local policies and procedures that are applicable to the care setting in which you are engaging in work experience or employment. It is good practice to ask your line manager about the existence and the whereabouts of the care setting's policies and procedures.

Key safeguarding points

+ 'All services must have a publicly declared "No Tolerance" approach to any form of abuse and must promote a culture which supports this ethos.'

+ Every individual has the right to a life free from abuse.

+ A culture of 'zero tolerance' of abuse must be fostered.

+ Safeguarding adults is everyone's responsibility.

+ Good multi-agency working is essential in line with local and national policy and procedures.

> **A vulnerable person is an adult who may be restricted in capacity to guard him/herself against harm or exploitation or to report such harm or exploitation.**
>
> (HSE, 2014.)

Harm or exploitation may occur as a result of physical and/or intellectual impairment. Due to a person's vulnerability, the individual may be in receipt of a care service in his or her own home, in the community or be resident in a residential care home, nursing home or other setting.

(Source: https://www.hse.ie/eng/about/who/socialcare/safeguardingvulnerableadults)

Vulnerable adults have the right:

+ to be accorded the same respect and dignity as any other adult, by recognising their uniqueness and personal needs

+ to be given access to knowledge and information in a manner which they can understand in order to help them make informed choices

+ to live safely without fear of violence in any form

+ to have their money, goods and possessions treated with respect and to receive equal protection for themselves and their property through the law

+ to be given guidance and assistance in seeking help because of abuse

+ to be supported in bringing a complaint

+ to have alleged, suspected or confirmed cases of abuse investigated promptly and appropriately

+ to receive support, education and counselling following abuse.

Barriers for the vulnerable adult to disclose abuse are:

+ fear on the part of the service user of having to leave their home or service

+ a lack of awareness that what they are experiencing is abuse

+ a lack of clarity as to whom they should talk

+ a lack of capacity to understand and report the incident

+ fear of an alleged abuser

+ limited verbal and other communication skills

+ fear of upsetting relationships

+ shame and/or embarrassment.

What to Do if an Older Person Reports an Alleged Concern to You

All cases of alleged or suspected abuse must be taken seriously.

✦ All staff must inform their line managers immediately if they have any concerns regarding allegations of abuse.

✦ All services must have effective mechanisms in place to ensure a prompt response to concerns and complaints.

✦ The safety and well-being of the vulnerable person is the priority consideration.

What is abuse?

Abuse may be defined as:

… any act, or failure to act, which results in a breach of a vulnerable person's human rights, civil liberties, physical and mental integrity, dignity or general well-being, whether intended or through negligence, including sexual relationships or financial transactions to which the person does not or cannot validly consent, or which are deliberately exploitative. Abuse may take a variety of forms.

(Source: National Council on Ageing and Older People (NCAOP), 2002.)

The age of sixty-five is taken as the point beyond which abuse may be considered to be elder abuse.

Types of abuse

There are seven types of abuse:

1 Physical abuse

2 Psychological abuse

3 Financial abuse

4 Sexual abuse

5 Neglect and acts of omission

6 Discrimination abuse

7 Institutional abuse.

HIQA and safe services standard

Theme 3: Safe Services Standard

+ Each resident is safeguarded from abuse and neglect.

+ The care service has effective plans in place to manage risk and protect residents from the risk of harm.

+ Each resident is protected through the care services policies and procedures.

+ Arrangements to protect residents from harm, promote bodily integrity, personal freedom and a restraint-free environment are in place.

+ Each resident's personal property and finances are managed and protected.

(HIQA, 2016.)

It is important to remember that elder abuse is an infrequent occurrence, but unfortunately, it does occur. An older person may experience more than one form of abuse at any given time. Healthcare professionals have a responsibility to be vigilant and to report any concerns they may have in relation to safeguarding the older person being cared for in a timely and appropriate manner.

Case Study: Mrs F

Health care assistant Ms B was assisting resident Mrs F with a shower, when she noticed that Mrs F had bruising to her arm. Health care assistant Ms B reported this to the nurse. Initially, Mrs F reported that she did not know how the bruise occurred. Later that day Mrs F broke down crying and shared the following information with health care assistant Ms B.

Mrs F is 76 years of age and only receives visits from her only nephew who is in his 40s; she has no other family alive and she indicates that she does not want to get her nephew into any trouble.

She states that on previous visits her nephew appeared short-tempered, had become verbally aggressive towards her and had asked her for money. Over the last few weeks this behaviour had escalated: he had become physically aggressive towards her. When Mrs F informed him that she did not have any money to give to him, he pushed her towards the chair, causing her to fall.

Although Mrs F is clear that 'this is out of the ordinary for him', she admits that she is afraid of him and is fearful that the behaviour could escalate.

Task Discuss and debrief on the case study outlined above:

1   Discuss in groups if there is abuse occurring in this situation.

2   Outline the types of abuse occurring.

3   Outline the steps you should take to keep Mrs F safe.

4   Outline the steps that the care setting could take to keep Mrs F safe.

5   Discuss if there are other stakeholders to be informed, for example, the guards, the resident's doctor, other staff members, HIQA.

chapter 21

POSITIVE LEISURE, RETIREMENT AND LIFELONG LEARNING

Positive leisure, retirement and lifelong learning opportunities are central components for the older person to age actively. In Ireland there are many different options available for the older person to enjoy in relation to leisure pursuits and lifelong learning. There are many benefits to be gained for the older person participating in pastimes, education and learning into their retirement. In previous chapters we learned that an older person's social needs are a very important part of their hierarchy of needs. Engaging in hobbies and activities has many

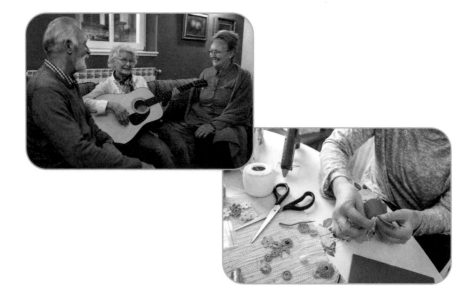

physical and psychological advantages. Additionally, the involvement in lifelong learning and education can have a positive influence with regard to the older person's self-esteem, with them reaching and maximising their potential. Their emotional well-being can also be enhanced. In Ireland there are a number of initiatives that promote leisure activities and attempt to make these pursuits more accessible for the older person.

Leisure Initiatives for the Older Person

The Positive Ageing Strategy

The aim of this strategy is to promote and maintain the participation of the older person in physical activity, which can also help to improve their mental health and well-being.

National Grant Scheme for Sport and Physical Activity for Older People

This scheme encourages older members of the community to participate in sport and physical activity. 'Go for Life' is an Age and Opportunity initiative funded by the Irish Sports Council that is run in cooperation with the HSE. It is a national programme for promoting physical activity in the older population.

(Age and Opportunity, 2015.)

Get Ireland Active

This is a public health campaign run by the HSE. The campaign aims to improve and encourage access to physical activity amenities by providing accessible information by geographic location on the type of leisure pursuits that are available from area to area.

(HSE, 2017.)

It is important that if an older person is approaching retirement age that they are advised in relation to the initiatives outlined above. As identified in previous chapters, the importance of retirement planning is paramount to facilitate a positive retirement process for the older person.

Moreover, the older person could be informed and encouraged to try a new hobby or pastime, to take up a new activity or engage in moderate intensity exercise. This can help the older person's acceptance of their retirement by offering continued structure, which can lead to an improved enjoyment of their retirement.

Education and Lifelong Learning

Education and lifelong learning creates new opportunities for the older person. It allows them to explore new concepts and opens up new opportunities in the world of work. Lifelong learning and education is a key part of Adult and Community Education. These educational initiatives provide a range of positive outcomes for the growing number of older people in Ireland, including an improved quality of life, reduced risk of isolation and social exclusion, an increase in self-esteem and self-confidence and a positive impact on general mental well-being. It can allow the older person to be socially active while learning new skills, which has benefits for cognitive health also.

Some research has been done amongst older people to determine how they felt about lifelong learning and how it impacted on their lives. These are some of the findings and recommendations:

+ 'I have found it a great way of meeting people of like mind and interests.'

+ 'Don't be afraid to start small. We were just a small group of people, most of whom had not previously met but who were interested in expanding their horizons. Now we have regular speakers, take field trips and go on overnight trips together.'

- ✚ 'I schedule summer visits and theatre trips. I refer to this as "me time".'

- ✚ 'Our activities and attitudes prove that we are more than our pathology or chronological age.'

- ✚ 'Communication is better than medication.'

(Source: https://www.ageaction.ie/how-we-can-help/lifelong-learning-u3a/what-members-say-about-u3a)

The Impact of Moving from Home to a Nursing Home

The process of leaving your home can be a difficult process for everyone. As the old saying goes, 'Home is where the heart is'. This is particularly so for the older person, whose home may have been a safe haven for them throughout their life. As a result, the change to a care environment can be difficult for the older person and can impact on their well-being. Healthcare professionals must be aware of this from the outset of providing care to an older person.

The governance and management of nursing homes have changed substantially over the past number of decades. These changes have occurred as a result of government policy and independent statutory bodies such as HIQA, who have developed and endorsed care standards and regulations. Furthermore, older people and their families who are seeking long-term care are more aware of what a high-quality service looks like, while their rights and their expectations of care services have also increased.

Nursing Homes Ireland is the national representative body for both private and voluntary nursing homes. Currently, there are over 460 nursing homes in Ireland providing care to over 25,000 people. The function of Nursing Homes Ireland is to proactively support and represent their nursing home members, facilitating them to provide sustainable, high-quality care to their residents.

(Source: Nursing Homes Ireland 2019. Source: https://nhi.ie)

Furthermore, an older person's decision to move to a nursing home illustrates the beginning of a new stage of their life journey. This change can carry with it anxiety and uncertainty. It is important to understand and to empathise with the older person that, the move from home to a nursing home can be daunting, but that the move can also open up a new way of living and opportunities to enhance holistic well-being.

Admission to the nursing home

For the older person who is admitted to a nursing home, it is important that they receive a positive admission. Some care settings will first provide a pre-admission, where they will visit the older person in their own home, in the hospital or the setting from which the older person will be admitted. This can help the older person to feel more comfortable and in control of their care, as the nursing home representative can begin to learn about their needs and wishes. This can enhance the process of admission to the care setting, so that care needs, care expectations and care equipment can be in place for the older person before they are admitted to the nursing home.

Healthcare professionals should be conscious to welcome the older person to the care setting. This introduction to the care setting can include:

+ an introduction to other residents and staff
+ a guided tour of their new home
+ a discussion where they are involved in the decisions made about their care, including care assessments and care plans.

The older person should have their voices heard: they should be actively listened to and staff should ask the older person questions about their own routines, their habits, their likes and dislikes, so that the transition to the nursing home can be as seamless as possible. It is also good practice to include the older person's next of kin or their representative in the process of their admission and in the completion of a person's individual care plan.

The Challenges Faced by the Older Person in Relation to Adapting to a New Environment

Task Working in groups, discuss some challenges you think an older person may face adapting to a new environment.

There is an acknowledgment that an older person may face challenges in relation to adapting to a new environment. The older person may find it difficult to accept that they require a level of assistance or an increased amount of help with their activities of daily living within a new environment. An older person may feel vulnerable, especially if they are not used to receiving assistance with personal grooming, personal hygiene and dressing. The vulnerability of this experience for an older person can be a challenge for them within any new care setting. An older person may also find it difficult to mobilise around an unfamiliar environment and this can impede a person's independence and their self-esteem. An older person may find it challenging to share a living space with other people; this may include a shared dining experience, a living room experience and/or a bedroom.

In addition, an older person may feel that they are losing their autonomy in relation to the care decisions and the care interventions they are receiving. An older person may have a longing for the home that they have made; they may miss the closeness of community spirit, the accessibility of family and friends and the local amenities that they have enjoyed.

Task Working in groups, discuss how you as a healthcare professional can enhance the transition from home to a new environment for the older person.

The Role of the All Ireland Gerontological Nurses Association

The All Ireland Gerontological Nurses Association of Ireland (AIGNA) is the voice of older people's nursing throughout Ireland. AIGNA represents nurses who work with older people across a range of healthcare settings. The association's main aim is to promote healthy ageing and the well-being of older people through excellence in gerontological nursing.

AIGNA offers master classes and conferences to nurses and allied healthcare professionals throughout the year. These master classes adhere to national and international best practice guidelines. They focus on different topics that are relevant to the care of the older person and provide education and learning opportunities to its members.

(Source: https://www.aigna.ie)

The Multidisciplinary Team

The role of the speech and language therapist

The speech and language therapist (SLT) works with an individual to manage any speech, language and/or communication difficulties. SLTs also assess and treat people who may have difficulty with eating, drinking and swallowing. SLTs work in different ways:

+ The SLT will support the person individually and talk to them about speech, language and/or communication needs. The SLT will then work with the individual to develop skills and strategies to allow the person to communicate meaningfully.

+ The SLT will also meet with the inner circle of family and friends including colleagues, other members of the multidisciplinary team, including doctors, nurses and health care assistants, to assist them in understanding how best to support the person's communication skills.

+ If an assessment of eating, drinking and swallowing ability is required, the SLT will meet the person to discuss how the assessment is carried out and how it can enhance a person's quality of life.

(Source: https://www.iaslt.ie/about/about_whatwedo.php)

The role of the physiotherapist

Physiotherapy, often referred to as physio, uses physical methods, such as massage and manipulation, to promote healing and well-being. Physiotherapy treatments are often used to help restore a person's range of movement after injury or illness.

Physiotherapists also help people with mental health conditions, neurological conditions (those affecting the brain and nervous system) and chronic (long-term) health conditions. For example, arthritis is a chronic condition that causes painful, stiff joints and is often associated with ageing. Physiotherapists can help keep the joints mobile and strengthen the surrounding muscles.

(Source: https://www.hse.ie/eng/health/az/p/physiotherapy/introduction.html)

The role of the occupational therapist

Occupational therapy aims to promote people's health and well-being through their ability to perform everyday activities of daily living with independence. The occupational therapist (OT) aims to facilitate the person to live more independently and with an advanced quality of life. They use techniques to improve a person's functional ability by changing or modifying their environment and/or equipment. They may also implement the use of assistive technologies.

(Source: https://www.hse.ie/eng/health/az/o/occupational-therapy/introduction.htm)

APPENDICES

INTAKE AND OUTPUT CHART

Name:			Date:		
Record for Intake			**Record for Output**		
Time	Intake Amount	Type of Intake	Time	Output Amount	Type of Output

MALNUTRITION UNIVERSAL SCREENING TOOL 'MUST'

 'Malnutrition Universal Screening Tool'

BAPEN
www.bapen.org.uk

BAPEN is registered charity number 1023927 www.bapen.org.uk

'MUST'

'MUST' is a five-step screening tool to identify **adults,** who are malnourished, at risk of malnutrition (undernutrition), or obese. It also includes management guidelines which can be used to develop a care plan.

It is for use in hospitals, community and other care settings and can be used by all care workers.

This guide contains:

- A flow chart showing the 5 steps to use for screening and management
- BMI chart
- Weight loss tables
- Alternative measurements when BMI cannot be obtained by measuring weight and height.

The 5 'MUST' Steps

Step 1
Measure height and weight to get a BMI score using chart provided. *If unable to obtain height and weight, use the alternative procedures shown in this guide.*

Step 2
Note percentage unplanned weight loss and score using tables provided.

Step 3
Establish acute disease effect and score.

Step 4
Add scores from steps 1, 2 and 3 together to obtain overall risk of malnutrition.

Step 5
Use management guidelines and/or local policy to develop care plan.

Please refer to *The 'MUST' Explanatory Booklet* for more information when weight and height cannot be measured, and when screening patient groups in which extra care in interpretation is needed (e.g. those with fluid disturbances, plaster casts, amputations, critical illness and pregnant or lactating women). The booklet can also be used for training. See *The 'MUST' Report* for supporting evidence. Please note that 'MUST' has not been designed to detect deficiencies or excessive intakes of vitamins and minerals and is of **use only in adults.**

Step 1 + Step 2 + Step 3

BMI score   **Weight loss score**   **Acute disease effect score**

BMI kg/m²	Score
>20 (>30 Obese)	= 0
18.5-20	= 1
<18.5	= 2

Unplanned weight loss in past 3-6 months

%	Score
<5	= 0
5-10	= 1
>10	= 2

If patient is acutely ill **and** there has been or is likely to be no nutritional intake for >5 days

Score 2

If unable to obtain height and weight, see reverse for alternative measurements and use of subjective criteria

Acute disease effect is unlikely to apply outside hospital. See 'MUST' Explanatory Booklet for further information

Step 4

Overall risk of malnutrition

Add Scores together to calculate overall risk of malnutrition
Score 0 Low Risk   Score 1 Medium Risk   Score 2 or more High Risk

Step 5

Management guidelines

0
Low Risk
Routine clinical care

- Repeat screening
  Hospital – weekly
  Care Homes – monthly
  Community – annually
  for special groups
  e.g. those >75 yrs

1
Medium Risk
Observe

- Document dietary intake for 3 days
- If adequate – little concern and repeat screening
  - Hospital – weekly
  - Care Home – at least monthly
  - Community – at least every 2-3 months
- If inadequate – clinical concern – follow local policy, set goals, improve and increase overall nutritional intake, monitor and review care plan regularly

2 or more
High Risk
Treat*

- Refer to dietitian, Nutritional Support Team or implement local policy
- Set goals, improve and increase overall nutritional intake
- Monitor and review care plan
  Hospital – weekly
  Care Home – monthly
  Community – monthly

* Unless detrimental or no benefit is expected from nutritional support e.g. imminent death.

All risk categories:
- Treat underlying condition and provide help and advice on food choices, eating and drinking when necessary.
- Record malnutrition risk category.
- Record need for special diets and follow local policy.

Obesity:
- Record presence of obesity. For those with underlying conditions, these are generally controlled before the treatment of obesity.

Re-assess subjects identified at risk as they move through care settings

See The 'MUST' Explanatory Booklet for further details and The 'MUST' Report for supporting evidence.

© BAPEN

Step 1 – BMI score (& BMI)

BAPEN
www.bapen.org.uk

Height (feet and inches)

	4'9½	4'10½	4'11	5'0	5'0½	5'1½	5'2	5'3	5'4	5'4½	5'5½	5'6	5'7	5'7½	5'8½	5'9½	5'10	5'11	5'11½	6'0½	6'1	6'2	6'3	6'3½	6'4½
170	80	78	76	74	72	70	68	66	65	63	62	60	59	57	56	55	54	52	51	50	49	48	47	46	45
169	79	77	75	73	71	69	68	66	64	63	61	60	58	57	56	55	53	52	51	50	49	48	47	46	45
168	79	77	75	73	71	69	67	66	64	62	61	60	58	57	55	54	53	52	51	50	49	48	47	46	45
167	78	76	74	72	70	69	67	65	64	62	61	59	58	56	55	54	53	52	50	49	48	47	46	45	44
166	78	76	74	72	70	68	66	65	63	62	60	59	57	56	55	54	52	51	50	49	48	47	46	45	44
165	77	75	73	71	70	68	66	64	63	61	60	58	57	56	54	53	52	51	50	49	48	47	46	45	44
164	77	75	73	71	69	67	66	64	62	61	60	58	57	55	54	53	52	51	50	48	47	46	45	44	44
163	76	74	72	71	69	67	65	64	62	61	59	58	56	55	54	53	51	50	49	48	47	46	45	44	43
162	76	74	72	70	68	67	65	63	62	60	59	57	56	55	54	52	51	50	49	48	47	46	45	44	43
161	76	74	72	70	68	66	64	63	61	60	58	57	56	54	53	52	51	50	49	48	47	46	45	44	43
160	75	73	71	69	67	66	64	63	61	59	58	57	55	54	53	52	50	49	48	47	46	45	44	43	43
159	75	73	71	69	67	65	64	62	61	59	58	56	55	53	52	51	50	49	48	47	46	45	44	43	42
158	74	72	70	68	67	65	63	62	60	59	57	56	55	53	52	51	50	48	47	46	45	44	43	42	42
157	74	72	70	68	66	65	63	61	60	58	57	56	54	53	52	50	49	48	47	46	45	44	43	42	42
156	73	71	69	68	66	64	62	61	59	58	57	55	54	53	52	50	49	48	47	46	45	44	43	42	41
155	73	71	69	67	65	64	62	61	59	58	56	55	54	52	51	50	49	48	47	45	44	43	42	41	41
154	72	70	68	67	65	63	62	60	59	57	56	55	53	52	51	50	49	48	46	45	44	43	42	42	41
153	72	70	68	66	65	63	61	60	58	57	56	54	53	52	51	49	48	47	46	45	44	43	42	41	41
152	71	69	68	66	64	62	61	59	58	57	55	54	53	51	50	49	48	47	46	45	44	43	42	41	40
151	71	69	67	65	64	62	60	59	58	56	55	54	52	51	50	49	48	47	46	45	43	43	41	40	40
150	70	68	67	65	63	62	60	59	57	56	54	53	52	51	50	48	47	46	45	44	43	42	42	41	40
149	70	68	66	64	63	61	60	58	57	56	54	53	52	50	49	48	47	46	45	44	43	42	41	40	40
148	69	68	66	64	62	61	59	58	56	55	54	52	51	50	49	48	47	46	45	44	43	42	41	40	39
147	69	67	65	64	62	60	59	57	56	55	53	52	51	50	49	47	46	45	44	43	42	41	40	40	39
146	68	67	65	63	62	60	58	57	56	54	53	52	51	49	48	47	46	45	44	43	42	41	40	40	39
145	68	66	64	63	61	60	58	57	55	53	51	50	49	48	47	46	45	44	43	42	41	40	39	39	22 12
144	68	66	64	62	61	59	58	56	55	54	51	50	49	48	46	45	44	43	43	42	41	40	39	38	22 9
143	67	65	64	62	60	59	57	56	54	53	52	51	49	48	47	46	45	44	43	42	41	40	40	39	22 7
142	67	65	63	61	60	58	57	55	54	53	52	50	49	48	47	46	45	44	43	42	41	40	39	39	22 5
141	66	64	63	61	59	58	56	55	54	52	51	50	49	47	46	45	44	43	42	41	40	39	39	38	22 3
140	00	04	62	61	59	58	56	55	53	52	51	50	48	47	46	45	44	43	42	41	40	39	38	37	22 1
139	65	63	62	60	59	57	56	54	53	52	50	49	48	47	46	45	44	43	42	41	40	39	38	37	21 12
138	65	63	61	60	58	57	55	54	53	51	50	49	48	47	46	45	44	43	42	41	40	39	38	37	21 10
137	64	63	61	59	58	56	55	54	52	51	50	49	47	46	45	44	43	42	41	40	39	38	38	37	21 8
136	64	62	60	59	57	56	54	53	52	51	49	48	47	46	45	44	43	42	41	40	39	38	37	36	21 6
135	63	62	60	58	57	55	54	53	51	50	49	48	47	46	45	44	43	42	41	40	39	38	37	36	21 4
134	63	61	60	58	57	55	54	52	51	50	49	47	46	45	44	43	42	41	40	40	39	38	37	36	21 1
133	62	61	59	58	56	55	53	52	51	49	48	47	46	45	44	43	42	41	40	39	38	38	37	36	20 13
132	62	60	59	57	56	54	53	52	50	49	48	47	46	45	44	43	42	41	40	39	38	37	36	35	20 11
131	61	60	58	57	55	54	52	51	50	49	48	46	45	44	43	42	41	40	39	38	38	37	36	35	20 9
130	61	59	58	56	55	53	52	51	50	48	47	46	45	44	43	42	41	40	39	38	38	37	36	35	20 7
129	61	59	57	56	54	53	52	50	49	48	47	46	45	44	43	42	41	40	39	38	37	36	35	34	20 4
128	60	58	57	55	54	53	51	50	49	48	46	45	44	43	42	41	40	39	38	37	36	35	35	34	20 2
127	60	58	56	55	54	52	51	50	48	47	46	45	44	43	42	41	40	39	38	37	36	35	34	34	20 0
126	59	58	56	55	53	52	50	49	48	47	46	45	44	43	42	41	40	39	38	37	36	36	35	34	33	19 12
125	59	57	56	54	53	51	50	49	48	46	45	44	43	42	41	40	39	39	38	37	36	35	34	34	33	19 10
124	58	57	55	54	52	51	50	48	47	46	45	44	43	42	41	40	39	38	37	37	36	35	34	33	19 7
123	58	56	55	53	52	51	49	48	47	46	45	44	43	42	41	40	39	38	37	36	36	35	34	33	19 5
122	57	56	54	53	51	50	49	48	46	45	44	43	42	41	40	39	39	38	37	36	35	35	33	32	19 3
121	57	55	54	52	51	50	48	47	46	45	44	43	42	41	40	39	38	37	37	36	35	34	33	32	19 1
120	56	55	53	52	51	49	48	47	46	45	44	43	42	41	40	39	38	37	36	35	35	34	33	32	18 13
119	56	54	53	52	50	49	48	47	45	44	43	42	41	40	39	38	38	37	36	35	34	33	33	32	18 10
118	55	54	52	51	50	48	47	46	45	44	43	42	41	40	39	38	37	36	36	35	34	33	33	32	31	18 8
117	55	53	52	51	49	48	47	46	45	44	42	41	40	40	39	38	37	36	35	35	34	33	32	32	31	18 6
116	54	53	52	50	49	48	46	45	44	43	42	41	40	39	38	37	37	36	35	34	33	33	32	31	18 4
115	54	53	51	50	48	47	46	45	44	43	42	41	40	39	38	37	36	35	35	34	33	33	32	31	18 2
114	53	52	51	49	48	47	46	45	43	42	41	40	39	39	38	37	36	35	34	33	33	32	31	30	17 13
113	53	52	50	49	48	46	45	44	43	42	41	40	39	38	37	36	35	34	33	33	32	31	31	30	17 11
112	53	51	50	48	47	46	45	44	43	42	41	40	39	38	37	36	35	34	33	32	32	31	30	30	17 9
111	52	51	49	48	47	46	44	43	42	41	40	39	38	38	37	36	35	34	33	32	32	31	30	29	17 7
110	52	50	49	48	46	45	44	43	42	41	40	39	38	37	36	36	35	34	33	32	31	30	30	29	17 5
109	51	50	48	47	46	45	44	42	41	40	39	38	38	37	36	35	34	33	32	32	31	30	30	29	17 2
108	51	49	48	47	46	44	43	42	41	40	39	38	37	37	36	35	34	33	33	32	31	31	30	29	17 0
107	50	49	48	46	45	44	43	42	41	40	39	38	37	36	35	35	34	33	32	31	31	30	29	28	16 12
106	50	48	47	46	45	44	42	41	40	39	38	38	37	36	35	34	33	33	32	31	31	30	29	28	16 10
105	49	48	47	45	44	43	42	41	40	39	38	37	36	35	34	34	33	32	32	31	30	29	28	28	16 7
104	49	47	46	45	44	43	42	41	40	39	38	37	36	35	34	34	33	32	31	31	30	29	28	28	16 5
103	48	47	46	45	43	42	41	40	39	38	37	36	36	35	34	33	33	32	31	30	29	29	28	27	16 3
102	48	47	45	44	43	42	41	40	39	38	37	36	35	34	34	33	32	31	31	30	29	29	28	28	27	16 1
101	47	46	45	44	43	42	41	40	39	38	37	36	35	35	34	33	32	32	31	30	30	29	28	27	27	15 13
100	47	46	44	43	42	41	40	39	38	37	36	35	35	34	33	33	32	32	31	30	30	29	28	28	27	27	15 10
	1.46	1.48	1.5	1.52	1.54	1.56	1.58	1.6	1.62	1.64	1.66	1.68	1.7	1.72	1.74	1.76	1.78	1.8	1.82	1.84	1.86	1.88	1.9	1.92	1.94

Weight (kg) (left axis)

Weight (stones and pounds) (right axis)

Height (m)

© BAPEN

Note : The black lines denote the exact cut off points (30,20 and 18.5 kg/m²), figures on the chart have been rounded to the nearest whole number.

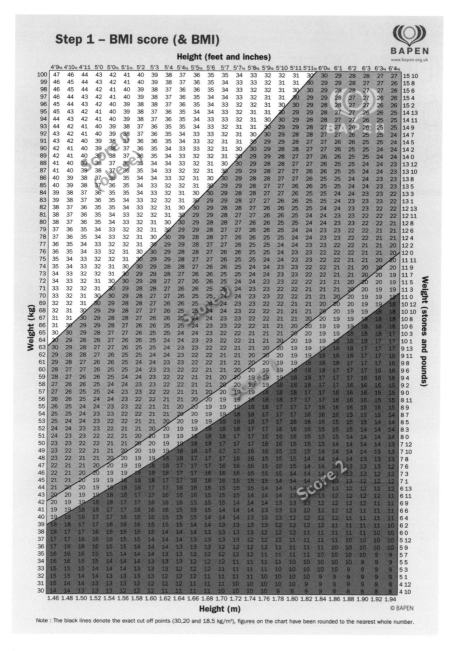

Note : The black lines denote the exact cut off points (30,20 and 18.5 kg/m²), figures on the chart have been rounded to the nearest whole number.

(Source: The 'Malnutrition Universal Screening Tool' ('MUST') is reproduced here with the kind permission of BAPEN (British Association for Parenteral and Enteral Nutrition). For further information on 'MUST' see www.bapen.org.uk. Copyright © BAPEN 2012)

IDDSI (INTERNATIONAL DYSPHAGIA DIET STANDARDISATION INITIATIVE)

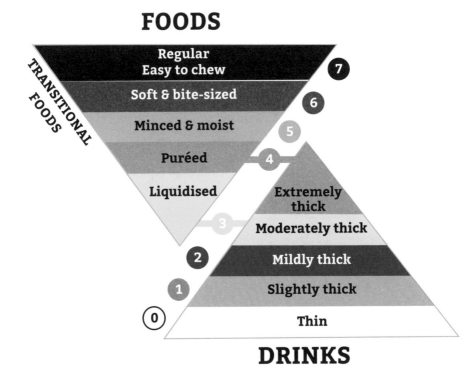

(Source: https://iddsi.org/)

THE BARTHEL SCALE

BARTHEL INDEX ACTIVITY	SCORE
FEEDING 0 = unable 5 = needs help cutting, spreading butter or may need modified diet 10 = independent	
BATHING 0 = dependent 5 = independent (bathing or showering)	
GROOMING 0 = needs help with personal care 5 = independent (face/hair/teeth/shaving – implements provided)	
DRESSING 0 = dependent 5 = needs help but can do about half unaided 10 = independent (including buttons/zips/laces)	
BOWELS 0 = incontinent (or needs enemas) 5 = occasional accident 10 = continent	
BLADDER 0 = incontinent or catheterised and unable to manage alone 5 = occasional accident 10 = continent	
TOILET USE 0 = dependent 5 = needs some help, but can do some things alone 10 = independent (on and off/dressing/wiping)	
TRANSFERS (BED TO CHAIR AND BACK) 0 = unable, no sitting balance 5 = major help (one or two people, physical), can sit 10 = minor help (verbal or physical) 15 = independent	
MOBILITY (ON LEVEL SURFACES) 0 = immobile or < 50 yards 5 = wheelchair independent, including corners > 50 yards 10 = walks with help one person (verbal or physical) > 50 yards 15 = independent (but may use any aid; for example, stick) > 50 yards	
STAIRS 0 = unable 5 = needs help (verbal, physical, carrying aid) 10 = independent	

QUESTION AND ANSWER SESSION

WITH A DIRECTOR OF CARE, STAFF NURSE AND A SENIOR HEALTH CARE ASSISTANT (HCA) IN RELATION TO PROVIDING HOLISTIC CARE

1 What are the most important qualities for a HCA to have when caring for an older adult?

Being a people person who can work with other people. Being adaptable and able to cope with the unexpected. Being able to remain calm in a challenging situation. Being able to cope with the stresses and strains in the personal lives and the health problems of the residents without being dragged down or becoming depressed by them. It's a job that can give lots of satisfaction, but it can also be very challenging, and you need to be able to manage those challenges. You also need to be a person who knows your limitations and who is willing to ask for help when needed. If you make a mistake, admit it. Don't try to cover up, because in healthcare, that could lead to greater problems arising. Nobody has all the answers – except teenagers, of course!

2 If you could offer one piece of advice to a newly qualified HCA, what would it be?

Be yourself. It's your greatest asset. There's nobody else like you. You are unique. People are not alike. Everybody is different. It doesn't work if you try to be somebody else. Personality is being yourself and that's what comes across to the people you care for and work with. A successful organisation harnesses the diverse talents of its entire staff.

3 What do you think are some of the challenges a HCA could face when caring for an older adult?

Remaining calm in dealing with a resident who displays aggressive and angry behaviour, and knowing how to keep you both safe.

Entering into the hallucinatory world of a resident suffering from dementia, similar to entering the imaginary world of a child.

There are also the obvious challenges involved in providing care, e.g. providing personal hygiene, etc.

4 What do you think are some of the positive aspects for a HCA in providing care for an older person?

Your world of work is full of change from minute to minute, hour to hour and day to day.

You can be part of a team involved in end-of-life care, enabling the resident's transition from this life to be as peaceful as possible. You also help the resident's family at this difficult time.

You are working as part of a caring team of colleagues and will form new friendships.

You become part of an organisation that is respected in the wider community for the work they do.

You will receive in-service training to further improve your caring skills.

5 **What opportunities do you think exist for a HCA caring for the older person?**

You may decide to pursue further studies in healthcare. Some HCAs go on to qualify as nurses or take up social studies.

In smaller, private nursing homes the opportunities for promotion are limited, but in public ones there are many such opportunities.

Further opportunities include working in home care and sheltered housing villages.

THE ABBEY PAIN SCORE

For measurement of pain in people with dementia who cannot verbalise.

How to use scale: While observing the resident, score questions 1 to 6.

Name of resident: _____

Name and designation of person completing the scale:

_____

Date: _____   **Time:** _____

Latest pain relief given was: _____at: _____hrs.

Q. 1   Vocalisation
e.g. whimpering, groaning, crying   Q. 1 [　]
Absent 0   Mild 1   Moderate 2   Severe 3

Q. 2   Facial expression
e.g. looking tense, frowning, grimacing, looking   Q. 2 [　]
frightened
Absent 0   Mild 1   Moderate 2   Severe 3

Q. 3   Change in body language
e.g. fidgeting, rocking, guarding part of body,   Q. 3 [　]
withdrawn
Absent 0   Mild 1   Moderate 2   Severe 3

Q. 4   Behavioural change

e.g. increased confusion, refusing to eat, alteration   Q. 4

in usual patterns

Absent 0   Mild 1   Moderate 2   Severe 3

Q. 5   Physiological change

e.g. temperature, pulse or blood pressure outside   Q. 5

normal limits, perspiring, flushing or pallor

Absent 0   Mild 1   Moderate 2   Severe 3

Q. 6   Physiological change

e.g. skin tears, pressure areas, arthritis, contractures,   Q. 6

previous injuries

Absent 0   Mild 1   Moderate 2   Severe 3

Add scores for 1–6 and record here   ➡   **Total Pain Score**

Now tick the box that matches the Total Pain Score

0–2	3–7	8–13	14+
No pain	Mild	Moderate	Severe

Finally, tick the box that matches the type of pain

Chronic	Acute	Acute on chronic

REFLECTIONS FROM A RETIRED COMMUNITY NURSE

1   **Having worked as a nurse in the community, can you list the main role of the home help within the home of an older person?**

The primary role of a home help within the home is to support the elderly client to remain in their own home for as long as possible and to provide assistance with basic everyday tasks.

2   **What are the benefits for health care assistants caring for the older person in their home?**

Knowing that you can make a difference to the individual's quality of life, providing companionship and building personal, yet professional, working relationships with clients and their families. This can guarantee a personally rewarding career for the healthcare worker.

3   **Reporting the well-being of the older person is a very important part of the role of the home help. As a nurse who has worked in the community, what do you think a home help should report back to the team?**

Any change in a client's condition that escalates concern will need to be reported without delay to one's line manager. Observance is one of the most essential qualities of the home help. By using one's eyes, ears, nose, touch and knowledge of what is normal for the person you care for, serious changes can be quickly identified. By reporting these changes, steps can be taken to address concerns swiftly and effectively.

REFERENCES

Age and Opportunity, 2015. 'Annual Report'. <https://ageandopportunity.ie/wp-content/uploads/2019/04/AgeOpportunityAnnualReport2015.pdf>

Central Statistics Office, 2013. 'Population and Labour Force Projections, 2016–2046'. <https://www.cso.ie/en/media/csoie/releasespublications/documents/population/2013/poplabfor2016_2046.pdf>

Clarke, K.A., Iphofen, R., 2008. 'The effects of failing to believe patients' experience of chronic pain'. *Nursing Times*. <https://www.nursingtimes.net/clinical-archive/pain-management/the-effects-of-failing-to-believe-patients-experience-of-chronic-pain-26-02-2008/>

Department of Health, 2019. 'Health in Ireland: Key Trends 2018'. <https://www.gov.ie/en/publication/2b3ade-health-in-ireland-key-trends-2018/>

————, 2014. 'The Irish National Dementia Strategy'. <https://www.hse.ie/eng/about/who/healthwellbeing/healthy-ireland/publications/irish-dementia-strategy-1-.pdf>

————, 2013. 'The National Positive Ageing Strategy'. https://www.gov.ie/en/publication/737780-national-positive-ageing-strategy

————, 2017. 'Population Ageing in Ireland: Projections 2002–2021'. <https://health.gov.ie/wp-content/uploads/2014/03/Population-Ageing-in-Ireland-Projections-2002-2021.pdf>

————, 16 June 2004, Department of Health https://www.gov.ie/en/publication/ae543e-population-ageing-in-ireland-projections-2002-2021/?referrer=/wp-content/uploads/2014/03/population-ageing-in-ireland-projections-2002-2021.pdf/)

Enable Ireland & the Disability Federation of Ireland, 2016. 'Assistive Technology for People with Disabilities and Older People: A Discussion Paper'. <https://www.enableireland.ie/sites/default/files/publication/AT%20Paper%20final%20version.pdf>

Health Information and Quality Authority (HIQA), 2017. 'Regulatory Guidance for Residential Services for Older People'. < https://www.hiqa.ie/sites/default/files/2017-01/Food-and-Nutrition-Guidance.pdf>

————, 2016a. 'Report of the review of nutrition and hydration care in public acute hospitals'. <https://www.hiqa.ie/reports-and-publications/key-reports-and-investigations/report-review-nutrition-and-hydration-care>

----, 2016b. 'Guidance on Dementia Care for Designated Centres for Older People'. <https://www.hiqa.ie/sites/default/files/2017-01/Dementia_Care-Guidance.pdf>

----, 2016c. 'National Standards for Residential Care Setting for Older People in Ireland'. <https://www.hiqa.ie/reports-and-publications/standard/current-national-standards-residential-care-settings-older-people>

----, 2012. 'A Guide to the National Standards for Safer Better Healthcare'. <https://www.hiqa.ie/sites/default/files/2017-01/Safer-Better-Healthcare-Guide.pdf>

Health Service Executive (HSE), 2019. '<https://www.hse.ie/eng/health/az/p/parkinson's-disease/treating-parkinson's-disease.html>

----, 2019. <https://www2.hse.ie/conditions/mental-health/clinical-depression/clinical-depression-diagnosis.html>

----, 2018. 'Nursing Homes Support Scheme Information Booklet'. <https://www2.hse.ie/file-library/fair-deal/nursing-homes-support-scheme-information-booklet.pdf>

----, 2017. 'Healthy Ireland Implementation Plan 2018–2022'. <https://www.hse.ie/eng/about/who/healthwellbeing/healthy-ireland/publications/community-healthcare-west-healthy-ireland-implementation-plan-2018-2022.pdf>

----, 2014. 'Safeguarding Vulnerable Persons at Risk of Abuse: National Policy & Procedures'. <https://www.hse.ie/eng/services/publications/corporate/personsatriskofabuse.pdf>

----, 2009. 'Health Services Intercultural Guide'. <https://www.hse.ie/eng/services/publications/socialinclusion/interculturalguide/>

Help the Aged, 2001. 'Policy Research Institute on Ageing and Ethnicity'. <https://www.scie.org.uk/publications/guides/guide15/selectedresearch/whatdignitymeans.asp>

Irish Heart Foundation, 2017. 'Step by Step Through Stroke: A Guide for Those Affected By Stroke and Their Carers'. <http://irishheart.ie/wp-content/uploads/2017/01/Step_by_Step_Through_Stroke_-_SEPA_ready.pdf>

Mahoney, F., & Barthel, D. (1965). Functional evaluation: The Barthel Index. Maryland State Medical Journal, 14, 56-61.

National Council on Ageing and Older People (NCAOP), 2002. 'Protecting our Future: Report of the Working Group on Elder Abuse'. <http://www.ncaop.ie/publications/research/reports/73_ProtectingourFuture.pdf>

Nursing and Midwifery Board of Ireland (NMBI), 2015. 'Working With Older People: Professional Guidance'. <https://www.nmbi.ie/NMBI/media/NMBI/working-with-older-people.pdf?ext=.pdf>

Pierce, et al., 2014. 'Prevalence and Projections of Dementia in Ireland, 2011–2046'. <https://www.genio.ie/system/files/publications/Dementia_Prevalence_2011_2046.pdf>

Robertson & Kenny, 2016. 'You're Only As Old As You Feel'. Findings from The Irish Longitudinal Study on Ageing (TILDA). < https://tilda.tcd.ie/publications/reports/>

United Nations, 2017. 'World Population Ageing'. <https://www.un.org/en/development/desa/population/publications/pdf/ageing/WPA2017_Highlights.pdf>

Ward, 2019. 'The Irish adult's transition to retirement – wellbeing, social participation and health-related behaviours'. Findings from The Irish Longitudinal Study on Ageing (TILDA). <https://tilda.tcd.ie/publications/reports/pdf/Report_Retirement.pdf>

World Health Organization (WHO), 2017. 'Global strategy and action plan on ageing and health'. <https://www.who.int/ageing/global-strategy/en/>

----. 'Global Health and Aging'. Accessed via: <https://www.who.int/ageing/publications/global_health.pdf>

----, 2002. 'Proposed working definition of an older person in Africa for the MDS Project'. < https://www.who.int/healthinfo/survey/ageingdefnolder/en/>

World Health Organization & World Bank, 2011. 'World Report on Disability'. https://www.enableireland.ie/report-0

INDEX

For my nieces and nephews, Aoibhinn, Donnchadh, Domhnall, Sadhbh, Éabha, Danial, Méabh, Peigi, Fiadh and Séan Óg.

To Mom, Dad, James and Bruno, thank you for your help and continued support. Special thanks to Nuala, Titus and Fiona for their time and advice.

"We don't stop playing because we grow old; we grow old because we stop playing." – **George Bernard Shaw**